I'M STILL HERE

Neuropsychiatric Comorbidities with HIV and Antiretroviral Therapy (ART)

Complications of Living with HIV

TJ Wicker M.H.A.

I'm Still Here
Neuropsychiatric Comorbidities with HIV
and Antiretroviral Therapy (ART)
Copyright © 2019 by TJ Wicker M.H.A.

All rights reserved. No part of this publication may be reproduced, distributed, or transmitted in any form or by any means, including photocopying, recording, or other electronic or mechanical methods, without the prior written permission of the author, except in the case of brief quotations embodied in critical reviews and certain other non-commercial uses permitted by copyright law.

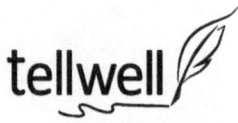

Tellwell Talent
www.tellwell.ca

ISBN
978-0-2288-1079-7 (Paperback)
978-0-22881-332-3 (eBook)

In dedication to my husband,
Jean Rock Claude St. Jacques

...... Tu seras toujours mon rayon de soleil,
même quand il y a des nuages!
Je t'aime de tout mon coeur......

TABLE OF CONTENTS

Preface vii

Chapter 1:	Introduction 1
Chapter 2:	Literature Review 13
Chapter 3:	Natural History 76
Chapter 4:	How to Test 84
Chapter 5:	CDC Classification 88
Chapter 6:	Antiretroviral (ART) History 90
Chapter 7:	The Early Days 108
Chapter 8:	Opportunistic Infections (OIs) 116
Chapter 9:	The Onset of Research 122
Chapter 10:	Theories 125
Chapter 11:	Mortality 131
Chapter 12:	A Widespread Global Pandemic 134
Chapter 13:	What are Antiretroviral Drugs and Antiretroviral Therapy (ART) 139
Chapter 14:	HIV Life Cycle 141
Chapter 15:	Approved Antiretroviral Drugs 144
Chapter 16:	HIV and Psychiatric Disorders 148
Chapter 17:	Psychiatric Manifestations with HIV and (ART) 162
Chapter 18:	HIV and Neurological Disorders 200
Chapter 19:	The US Aging Population with HIV 216
Chapter 20:	Data Collection Methods 222
Chapter 21:	Conclusion 236

List of Definitions 241
Drugs 265
References 285

PREFACE

BEGINNING IN the 1980s, *human immune deficiency virus* (HIV) infection emerged primarily as a rapidly progressive, unfamiliar death sentence, for which there was no treatment available. Later with the development of combination *antiretroviral therapy* (ART) in the mid-1990s, this transformed HIV, from a terminal death sentence, to a chronic manageable disease, despite the introduction, and usage of ART, significant numbers of patients continue to be affected by HIV-associated neurological, and psychiatric disorders.

CHAPTER 1

INTRODUCTION

I HOLD A particular interest in this topic, considering I have carried HIV for 32 years and have experienced, endured, and been treated for several neurological and psychiatric complications associated with my disease and the long-term effects of ART, even in lieu of the magnanimous recent advances with ART. July 2018, marked 32 years since the test that thrust me from one reality, into another. I was 23. I was astonished, confused, angry and tried very hard to register this in my head; why me? I told my partner at the time the news, who went and immediately got tested and learned he was negative. I told no one else, except for my Mother.

At this point in my life, my 32nd anniversary has me torn between disaffection and the bewildered realization that 30 plus years is ¾'s of my life. I became positive before some of my friends were even born. I have constantly reminded myself that for some bizarre reason, I never thought I'd live for so long. My survival has been dubiously uncertain, especially with my past continued drug addiction, severe depression and feeling hopeless, enough so, that I've never decided whether I should do anything serious with my life.

Now, mind you, I did go back to college, at age 48 and obtained a BSc in Public Service Administration & Policy and an MSc, in Healthcare Administration, which was without question, were my greatest accomplishments, especially considering I quit school at fifteen! This is not a biography of my life, (although, it is on my bucket list). The main purpose of this book, simply put, is to give a broad perspective of what it is like to live with the complications of HIV and ART. Throughout the greater part of my life, in lieu of just my disease, I have had to deal with survivor's guilt, which couples with long-term survivors, as most everyone I have known, got sick and died, while I have not.

Long-term survivors, such as myself, face many great challenges generally not shared by those diagnosed after 1996. Many of us continue to experience a cascade of physical symptoms, in part because we've spent years taking the "early drugs" that were either ineffective or harmful. Emotionally, we've suffered from the trauma of decades passing by, while watching our friends die painfully, while the entire time, expecting we would be next. At the beginning, no one knew long-term survival was even remotely possible, much less what it would look like.

I've seen enough people, men and women hit their 25th anniversary which is not so surprising anymore. We all have similar faces, we all know that this epidemiological global crisis is the most extraordinary one in modern times; we've seen the effects on science and sexuality. It's still not over; those awaiting treatment still outnumber those who have their disease under control. But the victory is still inevitable. We've done something with our lives. Ours and everyone else's.

The nurse's who drew our blood from the very first day, are now retiring. We'll continue to get older; we'll keep a pace with all those who are not positive. We'll hold back from dwelling on what we've lived through. We won't try and completely bore everyone commiserating about our condition. We'll have spared you. We won't have told you about the worst of it; most of us will have resorted to adages that are now truisms. The worst of AIDS hasn't been told. The books and films have been too afraid of scaring off our hard-won allies, and there's always that fear something worse will come along, a far more serious illness with less prospect of treatment. Victims of warfare and terrorist attacks and famine make us somehow look fortunate, so we've tried not to annoy you too much, even if some of us cashed in on our masochism.

Most people are totally unaware of the stringent medication regiment we have to go through. I began my HIV medication, in 1996, ten years after being diagnosed. I began with fourteen pills a day. Today, I take one pill per day, which has kept me from being undetectable for over 20 years. This repetition since 1996 has driven me crazy on the inside. Over these past 22 years, this fury has forced me into every single contortion I could possibly devise. I'm worn out by this constant compliance, even though I know anger and fatigue are pointless, it's my own prison, one that nobody can ever perceive or comprehend. I've come so far in my hatred that I take these tablets by myself, as if I were hiding this dismal reality. Now days, it has become a bit more acceptable to society, but at times, it's as if I want to shield everyone from this truism I've become.

Being HIV-positive changes you irrevocably, and these pills are the miracle workers that you have to show anybody who might claim it's not that serious to. Three hundred sixty-five days multiplied by 22 years makes 8,035 days I have taken medication in hopes that I will live a normal life. This doesn't convey just how exhausting this repetition has become. The worst part is that I'm actually grateful. These pills, some being quite toxic to certain individuals, have allowed me to live. My faith in medicine has continued to increase. Those dealing with health issues; skin, teeth, sight, heart, pre-mature aging, hearing, bones, guts and several other almost debilitating issues; I owe them my soundness of mind. But 32 years later, I'd never would have imagined it. I didn't want to die, but I didn't mean to live so long.

Over these 38 years, we've managed to slowly overpower this illness. But other conflicts have intensified in this time. A virulent virus turns out to have been easier to eradicate than colonialism or imperialism. Our environment is going to hell-and-a-hand-basket. Wars and attacks are flaring up everywhere. Famine is now compounded by drought, and all the rich just get richer and greedier. I've been thinking recently, that gay people ought to be happy, why not? But we're still a reminder of what has happened, of what we've endured. People abandon us one day or another, with just a text message and no explanation of why they don't want to see us ever again. We must keep quiet; we try and refrain from getting angry and we have to accept that we scare them since we're positive and, often, they're not.

Younger generations don't want to know anything, except what's in the now and are consumed with themselves; the millennials are the children of baby boomers, who are also known as the "Me Generation", who then produced the "Me Me Me Generation", whose selfishness technology and narcissistic attitude has only exacerbated.

In my own words, I find them to be socially retarded; it's quite sad that they live in a box of their own and have little interest of what the world has to offer, except for their own entitlement. The older ones are ashamed of their past, and the rest of us are dying off, all of us wellsprings of knowledge with thousands of stories to tell, but nobody is listening. All that's left are these pills that we hide and don't talk about.

There are neurological and psychiatric *comorbidities* that arise for those who live with HIV, whether patients are either on, or off ART. Being in healthcare off, and on, for several years, my interest in this global pandemic is both personal, and professional. There are newly diagnosed cases of HIV every day, in every corner of the world, and I believe with continued research, it could eventually save tens of thousands of lives.

Currently, the life expectancy of people with HIV has dramatically increased with recent advances in ART. The first known cases of HIV-related infections, of the unfamiliar disease, were reported in 1981. Along with more painstaking research, the virus was then identified as HIV, two years later, and almost immediately neurologic complications were recognized at a very early stage with this epidemic.

Furthermore, neuropsychiatric manifestations, and symptoms still remain prevalent since the earliest reports of HIV. The earliest neuropsychiatric manifestations documented by the very first reports included dementia, depression, psychomotor slowing, neurocognitive deficits, in addition to mania, and atypical psychosis. Initially, researchers believed these mental disturbances were attributed to the psychological reaction to contracting this disease itself.

Severe depression is by far one of the most common psychiatric disorders observed in all persons infected with HIV. Statistics have proven a wide variation, with 4% to 22% for HIV-*seropositive* men, and 2% to 18% for HIV-seropositive women. Major episodes of mania have also been documented with the progression of HIV infection. In the early stages of HIV infection, 1%–2% of patients experienced manic episodes, which is only slightly higher than the rate of the general population. Psychosis has also been highly documented, relative to the mood disorders, and uncommon psychiatric manifestations of having AIDS. Even with the implementation of antiretroviral therapy, it still may precipitate common episodes of psychosis.

AIDS-related complications of the *central nervous system* (CNS) can be caused directly by the HIV virus itself, especially in older persons, by certain cancers and opportunistic infections, (illnesses caused by fungi bacteria, and other viruses, or by toxic effects of the drugs used to treat these symptoms.) *AIDS HIV-associated dementia* (HAD), and *AIDS-dementia complex* (ADC), occurs primarily in persons with advanced HIV infection. Symptoms may include *encephalitis* (inflammation of the brain), behavioral changes, and a slow but gradual decline in cognitive function, including trouble with concentration, memory, and attention. *Cryptococcal meningitis* is also prevalent in about 10% of untreated individuals with AIDS. *Herpes virus* infections are often seen in people with HIV. People with HIV/AIDS may suffer from several different forms of *neuropathy,* or nerve pain, and infected adults older than 50 years old represent more than 10% of the HIV-infected population, and 15% of all people living with AIDS. *Progressive multifo-*

cal leukoencephalopathy (PML) may also affect individuals with a compromised immune system including 5% of people with AIDS. Psychological and neuropsychiatric disorders can also occur at different phases of the HIV infection.

No single treatment can cure the neurological complications of HIV/AIDS. Some of these disorders require aggressive therapy, while others simply are treated symptomatically. Advances in *highly active antiretroviral therapy* (HAART) aims to improve the efficacy of HIV drugs as well as the quality of life in HIV-infected patients. Neurologic and psychological disturbances that occur because of HIV disease and therapy are of great concern, because they can overlap, and are often difficult to distinguish and their pathogenesis is not clearly understood.

Furthermore, these complications can lead to decreased medication adherence, thereby interfering with treatment outcomes. Antiretrovirals, including *nonnucleoside reverse transcriptase inhibitors* (NNRTIs), proved to penetrate the *central nervous system* (CNS), and suppress the viral replication, but they can also exacerbate CNS side effects and neuropsychiatric symptoms.

Although the correlations with neuropsychiatric symptoms, *neuroendocrine peptides* and the immune system still remains to be unclear and the emergence of neuropsychiatric complications during the course of HIV/AIDS still have serious effects when not identified quickly. Whether these complications are due to the direct or indirect effects of HIV on the brain, or to the effects of stress and depression, careful diagnosis and treatment are of the utmost importance. With further research, and investigation to try and elucidate potential causal mechanisms, holds the promise of refining existing therapies and the development of new treatment options.

The general problem is, since the onset of this global pandemic, there is an estimated 78 million people who have become infected with HIV, and an estimated 2.1 million individuals worldwide became newly infected with HIV in 2015, and 35 million people have died of AIDS-related illnesses. Even with combined understanding of HIV, its prevention, and treatment, there is still no cure. However, treatment with antiretroviral drugs can control the virus, but there is also a need to assist the neurological and psychiatric complications that are in conjunction with the disease.

Another specific problem is, even after years of improving antiretroviral therapy, neuropsychiatric complications still occur in as many as 50% of people living with HIV, in addition to a large percentage of older *long-term survivors*, like myself. Managing the mental disorders is also a crucial part of effective HIV/AIDS intervention program. Physicians and psychiatrists now must be familiar with disorders that are prevalent in HIV infection. There is estimation that 40–70% of patients with AIDS develop clinical neurological and psychiatric abnormalities.

Within this book, I will attempt to determine whether a relationship exists between having HIV, antiretroviral therapy, and the challenges physician's, psychiatrist's and pharmacological interactions face, with the different diagnosis's, the onset of neuropsychiatric comorbidities and non-classical presentations of common disorders that come with the management of HIV.

CHAPTER 2

LITERATURE REVIEW

I HAVE WRITTEN this book to offer my readers, a simple, concise overview of: What is HIV, how widespread is the disease, what is antiretroviral therapy ART and the neurological and psychiatric comorbidities that couple with having HIV and long-term antiretroviral therapy. The contents convey existing research to discuss these topics in detail, as to the significance and importance of this topic. It will also identify any gaps, weaknesses, controversies, and/or problems in the theories, the anatomy, etiology, physiology, and pathophysiology of the disease. Although past, and current literature covers a wide variety of theories, it will also focus on certain major concepts, which emerge repeatedly throughout the literature being reviewed.

What is HIV and how Widespread is the Disease?

Human immunodeficiency virus (HIV) is virus that attacks the body's immune system, the body's built in defense again illness and infection, leaving it vulnerable to several opportunistic infections and cancers. HIV is a blood borne pathogen present in bodily fluids, such as (blood, semen, including pre-cum, rectal fluid, vaginal fluid and in breast milk. The virus destroys our white blood cells in the immune system, which are called T-helper cells, also called (CD-4 cells), and it makes copies of itself, and multiplies inside the T-cells, which, without treatment, will become more difficult for the body to fight off any infections or other diseases. If HIV goes untreated, it could take up to 10 to 15 years, before for the immune system is so severely damaged, that it can no longer can defend itself at all. However, the speed HIV progresses will vary depending on the age of the person, their health and background.

The pandemic of the human immunodeficiency virus HIV disease, eventually resulting in *acquired immune deficiency syndrome* (AIDS), is currently the most important public health event in recent history, with epic proportions that has political, social, economic, and cultural implications far beyond its medical significance. June 5, 1981, marks the official point zero of the human immunodeficiency virus HIV epidemic. On that date, the *Centers for Disease Control and Prevention* (CDC) published what has become a landmark communication in its *Morbidity and Mortality Weekly Report* (MMWR).

Timeline of HIV (37 Years of AIDS)

The following timeline of HIV, I find to be pertinent to my subject, which documents the magnanimous advances technology has made with trying to eradicate HIV.

1981

On June 5, the U.S. *Centers for Disease Control and Prevention* (CDC) published a Morbidity and Mortality Weekly Report (MMWR) describing cases of a new rare lung infection, *Pneumocystis carinii pneumonia* (PCP), in five young, previously healthy, gay men in Los Angeles. All the men have other unusual infections as well, indicating that their immune systems are not working; two have already died by the time the report is published. This edition of the MMWR marks the first official reporting of what will become known as the AIDS epidemic. By year-end, there are a cumulative total of

270 reported cases of severe immune deficiency among gay men, and 121 of those individuals have died.

1982

The City and County of San Francisco, working closely with the Shanti Project and the San Francisco AIDS Foundation, develop the "San Francisco Model of Care," which emphasized home and community-based services. On April 13, U.S. Representative Henry Waxman convenes the first congressional hearings on HIV/AIDS. The (CDC) estimates that tens of thousands of people may be affected by the disease. On September 24, CDC uses the term "AIDS" (acquired immune deficiency syndrome) for the first time and releases the first case definition of AIDS: "a disease at least moderately predictive of a defect in cell-mediated immunity, occurring in a person with no known case for diminished resistance to that disease."

1983

On January 7th, the CDC reports cases of AIDS in female sexual partners of males with AIDS. In February, Dr. Robert Gallo, from the *National Institutes of Health* (NIH), suggests that a retrovirus causes AIDS. In the March 4th edition of the *Morbidity and Mortal-*

ity Weekly Report (MMWR), CDC notes that most cases of AIDS have been reported among homosexual men having sex with multiple sexual partners, injection drug users, Haitians and hemophiliacs. The report suggests that AIDS may be caused by an infectious agent that is transmitted sexually or through exposure to blood or blood products and issues recommendations for preventing transmission. On May 20th, Professor Luc Montagnier, of the Pasteur Institute in France, reports the discovery of a retrovirus named *Lymphadenopathy Associated Virus* (LAV) that could be the cause of AIDS. On July 25th, San Francisco General Hospital opens the first dedicated AIDS ward in the U.S. It becomes fully occupied within days. In the September 9th MMWR, CDC identifies all major routes of HIV transmission and rules out transmission by casual contact, food, water, air or environmental surfaces.

1984

The Long Island AIDS Project (LIAP) started the first AIDS Family and Bereavement Support Groups on Long Island. Community-based AIDS service organizations join together to form AIDS Action, a national organization in Washington, DC, to advocate on behalf of people and communities affected by this epidemic and to educate the Federal Government, and to help shape AIDS-related policy and legislation. In June, Dr. Gallo and Professor Luc Montagnier, from the Pasteur Institute in France, held a joint press conference to announce that Dr. Montagnier's Lymphadenopathy Associated Virus (LAV) and Dr. Gallo's HTLV-III virus are certainly identical and are the likely cause of AIDS.

1985

LIAP starts the first support group for people with AIDS. Ryan White, an Indiana teenager who contracted AIDS through contaminated blood products used to treat his hemophilia, is refused entry to his middle school. He goes on to speak publicly against AIDS stigma and discrimination. On January 11th, the CDC revises the AIDS case definition to note that AIDS is caused by a newly identified virus and issues provisional guidelines for blood screening. Actor Rock Hudson dies of AIDS-related illness on October 2nd. Hudson leaves $250,000 to help set up the *American Foundation for AIDS research* (amfAR). Elizabeth Taylor served as the founding National Chairman. At least one HIV case has been reported from each region of the world.

1986

On January 16th, The CDC reports that more people were diagnosed with AIDS in 1985 than in all earlier years combined. The 1985 figures show an 89% increase in new AIDS cases compared with 1984. Of all AIDS cases to date, 51% of adults and 59% of children have died. The new report shows that, on average, AIDS patients die about 15 months after the disease is diagnosed. Public health experts predict twice as many new AIDS cases in 1986.

Four months later, the International Committee on the Taxonomy of Viruses announces that the virus that causes AIDS will officially be known as "Human Immunodeficiency Virus" (HIV).

July 18th, at the *National Conference on AIDS in the Black Community* in Washington, DC, a group of minority leaders meets with the U.S. Surgeon General, Dr. C. Everett Koop, to discuss concerns about HIV/AIDS in communities of color. This meeting marks the unofficial founding of the National Minority AIDS Council.

In October of this year, the Robert Wood Johnson Foundation creates the *AIDS Health Services Program*, providing $17.2 million in funding for patient-care demonstration projects in 11 cities. The goal is to replicate the San Francisco Model of Care nationwide—but with an emphasis on tailoring programs to meet the needs in local contexts.

Later this month, the U.S. *Health Resources and Services Administration* (HRSA) begins its AIDS Service Demonstration Grants program—the agency's first AIDS-specific health initiative. In the program's first year, HRSA makes $15.3 million available to four of the country's hardest-hit cities: New York, San Francisco, Los Angeles, and Miami.

Then, in late October, the Surgeon General issues the *Surgeon General's Report on AIDS* . The report makes it clear that HIV cannot be spread casually and calls for: a nationwide education campaign (including early sex education in schools); increased use of condoms; and voluntary HIV testing.

Two days later in October, the CDC reports that AIDS cases are disproportionately affecting African Americans and Latinos. This is particularly true for African American and Latinx children, who make up 90% of perinatally acquired AIDS cases.

Then on October 29th, the *Institute of Medicine* (IOM), the principal health unit of the National Academy of Sciences, issues a report, *Confronting AIDS: Directions for Public Health, Health Care, and Research*

. The report calls for a "massive media, educational and public health campaign to curb the spread of the HIV infection," as well as for the creation of a National Commission on AIDS. The IOM estimates that the effort will require a $2 billion investment in research and patient care by the end of the decade.

1987

LIAAC was asked to facilitate workshops at the National Lesbian and Gay Health Conference/Fifth National AIDS Forum in Los Angeles. Emmy-award winning pianist, Liberace, dies of AIDS-related illness on February 4th. On March 19th, the U.S. *Food and Drug Administration* (FDA) approves the first antiretroviral drug, *zidovudine* (AZT). The U.S. Congress approves $30 million in emergency funding to states for AZT, laying the groundwork for what will be the *AIDS Drug Assistance Program* (ADAP), authorized by the Ryan White CARE Act in 1990.

In April, the FDA approves the Western blot blood test kit, a more specific test for HIV antibodies. In May, the FDA creates a new class of experimental drugs, Treatment Investigational New Drugs, which accelerates drug approval by 2-3 years. On May 16th, the U.S. Public Health Service adds HIV as a "dangerous contagious disease" to its immigration exclusion list and mandated testing for all visa applicants. In October, the AIDS Memorial Quilt is displayed for the first time on the National Mall in Washington, DC. The display features 1,920 4"x 8" panels and drew over a half a million visitors. In October, AIDS becomes the first disease ever debated on the floor of the *United Nations* (UN) General Assembly. The General Assembly resolves to mobilize the entire UN system in the worldwide struggle against AIDS and designates the *World Health Organization* (WHO) to lead the effort

1988

The World Health Organization, WHO declares December 1st, to be the first World AIDS Day. Ryan White, an HIV-positive teenager who has become a national spokesperson for AIDS education, treatment, and funding, testifies before the President's Commission on AIDS. Elizabeth Glaser, an HIV-positive mother of two HIV-positive children, and two of her friends form the Pediatric AIDS Foundation (later renamed the Elizabeth Glaser Pediatric AIDS Foundation) advocate for research into the care and treatment needs of children living with HIV/AIDS. In April, the first comprehensive *needle-exchange program* (NEP) in North America is established in Tacoma, WA. San Francisco then follows and establishes what becomes the largest NEP in the nation.

1989

Photographer Robert Mapplethorpe dies of AIDS-related illness on March 9th, On June 23rd, CDC releases the Guidelines for Prevention of Transmission of Human Immunodeficiency Virus and Hepatitis B Virus to Health-Care and Public-Safety Workers. The U.S. *Health Resources and Services Administration* (HRSA) grants $20 million for HIV care and treatment through the Home-Based and Community-Based Care State grant program. For many states, this is their first involvement in HIV care and treatment. The number of reported AIDS cases in the United States reaches 100,000.

1990

LIAAC debuts its first original publication "Did You Think You Were Safe in the Suburbs?" On January 18th, the U.S. CDC reported the possible transmission of HIV to a patient through a dental procedure performed by an HIV-positive dentist. This episode provoked much public debate about the safety of common dental and medical procedures. Pop artist Keith Haring dies of AIDS-related illness on February 16th, and just two months later on April 8th, Ryan White died of AIDS-related illness at the age of 18. In July, the U.S. Congress enacts the *Americans with Disabilities Act* (ADA).

The Act prohibits discrimination against individuals with disabilities, including people living with HIV/AIDS. In August, the U.S. Congress enacts the Ryan White *Comprehensive AIDS Resources Emergency* (CARE) Act of 1990, which provides $220.5 million in Federal funds for HIV community-based care and treatment services in its first year. HRSA manage the program, which was the nation's largest HIV-specific Federal grant program. On October 26th, FDA approves use of AZT for pediatric AIDS.

1991

LIAAC Golf and Tennis Open is established. AIDS WALK Long Island is established. The Visual AIDS Artists Caucus launches the Red Ribbon Project to create a visual symbol to demonstrate compassion for people living with AIDS and their caregivers. The red ribbon become the international symbol of AIDS awareness. On July 21st, the CDC recommend restrictions on the practice of HIV-positive healthcare workers and Congress enacts a law requiring states to adopt the CDC restrictions or to develop and adopt their own.

On November 7th, American basketball star Earvin "Magic" Johnson announces that he was HIV-positive. Three weeks later, on November 24th, Freddie Mercury, lead singer/songwriter of the rock band Queen, dies of bronchial pneumonia resulting from AIDS, ironically enough, his death was one day after he publicly "came-out".

1992

The *New York State Department of Health* (NYSDOH) AIDS Institute awards *The Long Island Association for AIDS Care* (LIAAC) funding to establish our Nutrition for Life meals program, adding home delivery of nutritious meals to our services for our clients who are either at nutritional or financial risk. AIDS becomes the number one cause of death for U.S. men ages 25 to 44. On May 27th, the FDA licensed a 10-minute diagnostic test kit which could be used by health professionals to detect the presence of HIV-1. Florida teenager Ricky Ray dies of AIDS-related illness on December 13th. The 15-year-old hemophiliac and his two younger brothers sparked a national conversation on AIDS after their court battle to attend school led to boycotts by local residents and the torching of their home.

1993

LIAAC's Recovery Outreach Peer Program was established and The Community Follow-Up Program was also established, adding Medicaid reimbursed case management to LIAAC's services. LIAAC is featured in a New York Times article, "AIDS Care on the East End," highlighting the *Nutrition for Life* program as well as our support groups. President Clinton then establishes the White House *Office of National AIDS Policy* (ONAP). World-renowned ballet dancer Rudolf Nureyev dies of AIDS-related illness on January 6th, and tennis star Arthur Ashe dies on February 3rd. On May 7th, the FDA approved the first female condom. On December 18th, the CDC expanded the case definition of AIDS, declaring those with CD4 counts below 200 to have AIDS. In that same MMWR, CDC adds three new conditions; pulmonary tuberculosis, recurrent pneumonia, and invasive cervical cancer, to the list of clinical indicators of AIDS. These new conditions, they had believed, meant that more women and injection drug users will be diagnosed with AIDS.

1994

LIAAC partners with NYS AIDS Institute to co-sponsor the first Long Island "HIV/AIDS Bereavement Conference" for health care providers. AIDS becomes the leading cause of death for all Americans ages 25 to 44. On February 17th, Randy Shilts, a U.S. journalist who covered the AIDS epidemic and who authored "And the Band Played On: Politics, People, and the AIDS Epidemic", which were both fantastic books, dies of AIDS-related illness at age 42. On December 23rd, the FDA approves an oral HIV test, which was the first non-blood-based antibody test for HIV. The U.S. *Department of Health and Human Services* (HHS) issues guidelines requiring applicants for grants from the NIH to address, the appropriate inclusion of women and minorities in clinical research.

1995

Long Island Crisis Center names LIAAC's President and CEO, Dr. Gail Barouh, "Person of the Year." On February 23rd, Greg Louganis, Olympic gold medal diver, disclosed to the world, that he was HIV-positive. In June, the FDA approves the first protease inhibitor. This ushers in a new era of HAART. President Clinton establishes his *Presidential Advisory Council on HIV/ AIDS* (PACHA). The Council meets for the first time on July 28th. On September 22nd, the CDC reviews syringe exchange programs in the U.S, 1994-1995. The National Academy of Sciences concluded that syringe exchange programs 1995 should be regarded as an effective component of a comprehensive strategy to prevent infectious disease. By the end of that year, 500,000 cases of AIDS had been reported in the U.S.

1996

LIAAC sponsored community forums and advocated for the passage of the Managed Care Bill of rights. In Vancouver, the 11th International AIDS Conference highlights the effectiveness of HAART, creating a short period of optimism. The number of new AIDS cases diagnosed in the U.S. declines for the first time since the beginning of the epidemic. In 1996, within four short months, The FDA approved:

- The first HIV home testing and collection kit (May 14th)
- A viral load test, which measured the level of HIV in the blood (June 3rd)

- The first non-nucleoside reverse transcriptase inhibitor (NNRTI) drug, *nevirapine* (June 21st)— This would be the first antiretroviral drug I was given, in addition to AZT, after already being positive for ten years.
- The first HIV urine test (August 6th)

1997

LIAAC establishes The New York to the Hamptons Challenge Bike Ride. Later, in response to the call to "hit early, hit hard," HAART become the new standard of HIV care. The CDC reported the first substantial decline in AIDS deaths in the United States. Due to the use of HAART, AIDS-related deaths in the U.S. decline by 47% compared with the previous year. UNAIDS (the *Joint United Nations Programme on AIDS*) estimated that 30 million adults and children worldwide had HIV, and that, each day, 16,000 people become newly infected with the virus. As a greater number of people begin taking protease inhibitors, resistance to the drugs becomes more common, and drug resistance emerges as an area of grave concern within the AIDS community.

1998

LIAAC's Consumer Advisory Council is established. CDC reported that African Americans account for 49% of U.S. AIDS-related deaths. AIDS-related mortality for African Americans is 10 times that of Whites and three times that of Hispanics. With the leadership of the *Congressional Black Caucus* (CBC), Congress funds the Minority AIDS Initiative. An unprecedented $156 million is invested to improve the nation's effectiveness in preventing and treating HIV/AIDS in African American, Hispanic, and other minority communities. On April 24th, CDC issued the first national treatment guidelines for the use of antiretroviral therapy in adults and adolescents with HIV.

On June 25th, the U.S. Supreme Court rules that the ADA covered those in the earlier stages of HIV disease, not just those who had developed AIDS. On November 12th, the U.S. Congress enacts the Ricky Ray Hemophilia Relief Fund Act, honoring the Florida teenager who was infected with HIV through the transmission of contaminated blood products. The Act authorizes payments to individuals with hemophilia and other blood clotting disorders who were infected with HIV by unscreened blood-clotting agents between 1982 and 1987.

1999

LIAAC is central to the implementation of the NYSDOH, HIV reporting and partner notifications regulations on Long Island. WHO announces that HIV/AIDS has become the fourth biggest killer worldwide and the number one killer in Africa. WHO estimated that 33 million people are living with HIV worldwide, and that 14 million have died of AIDS. In March, VaxGen, a San Francisco-based biotechnology company, begins conducting the first human vaccine trials in a developing country, Thailand. On December 10th, the CDC released a new HIV case definition to help state health departments expand their HIV surveillance efforts and more accurately track the changing course of this pandemic.

2000

LIAAC sponsors the world's largest "Living AIDS Awareness Ribbon" in honor of year 2000. On April 30th, President Clinton declares that HIV/AIDS is a threat to U.S. national security. On May 10th, President Clinton issues an Executive Order to assist developing countries in importing and producing generic HIV treatments. Two-thousand more continued in August, the U.S. Congress enacted the Global AIDS and Tuberculosis Relief Act of 2000. In September, as part of its Millennium Declaration, the United Nations adopted the Millennium Development Goals which included a specific goal of reversing the spread of HIV/AIDS, malaria and TB. In October, the U.S. Congress reauthorized the Ryan White CARE Act for the second time.

2001

LIAAC receives its first Federal grant from The *Substance Abuse and Mental Health Service Administration* (SAMHSA). *The Center for Substance Abuse Treatment* (CSAT). February 7th marked the first annual National Black HIV/AIDS Awareness Day in the U.S. Newly appointed U.S. Secretary of State, Colin Powell, reaffirms the U.S. statement that HIV/AIDS is a national security threat. After generic drug manufacturers offer to produce discounted, generic forms of HIV/AIDS drugs for developing countries, several major pharmaceutical manufacturers agree to offer further reduced drug prices to those countries. The CDC announced a new HIV Prevention Strategic Plan to cut annual HIV infections in the U.S. by half within five years.

2002

On June 25th, the United States announced a framework that would allow poor countries, unable to produce pharmaceuticals to gain greater access to drugs which were needed to combat HIV/AIDS, malaria, and other public health issues. In July, UNAIDS (the *Joint United Nations Programme on AIDS*) reported that HIV/AIDS is now by far the leading cause of death in sub-Saharan Africa, and the fourth biggest global killer. The average life expectancy in sub-Saharan Africa falls between 47 years to 62 years as a result of AIDS. On November 7th, the FDA approved the first rapid HIV diagnostic test kit for use in the United States that provided results with 99.6 percent accuracy in as little as 20 minutes. Unlike other antibody tests for HIV, this new blood test could be stored at room temperature and required no specialized equipment and may be used outside of the traditional laboratory or clinical settings, allowing more widespread use of HIV testing. Worldwide, 10 million young people, aged 15-24 and three million children under 15 are living with HIV. During this year, 3.5 million new infections continued to occur in sub-Saharan Africa, and the epidemic will claim the lives of an estimated 2.4 million Africans.

2003

LIAAC purchases its first mobile van, utilized for mobile outreach, HIV testing and immediate linkages to substance abuse treatment. The CDC calculated that 27,000 of the estimated 40,000 new infections that occur each year in the U.S. resulted from transmission by individuals who do not know they are infected. On February 24th, VaxGen, a San Francisco-based biotechnology company, announces that its AIDSVAX vaccine trial failed to reduce overall HIV infection rates among those who were vaccinated. On April 18th, the CDC announced Advancing HIV Prevention: New Strategies for a Changing Epidemic, a new prevention initiative that aimed to reduce barriers to early diagnosis and increase access to, and utilization of, quality medical care, treatment, and ongoing prevention services for those living with HIV. October 15th marked the first annual *National Latino AIDS Awareness Day* (NALLD) in the U.S. On December 1st, WHO announced the "3 by 5" initiative, to bring treatment to 3 million people by 2005.

2004

Agency awarded its first CDC grant, expanding our HIV testing capability and introducing rapid testing to Long Island. On March 26th, the FDA approved the use of oral fluid samples with a rapid HIV diagnostic test kit that provided the result in 20 minutes. On June 10th, leaders of the *"Group of Eight"* (G8) Summit (Canada, France, Germany, Italy, Japan, Russia, the United Kingdom, and the United States) call for the creation of a *"Global HIV Vaccine Enterprise,"* a consortium of Government and private-sector groups designed to coordinate and accelerate research efforts to find an effective HIV vaccine.

2005

Agency established a new headquarters in a 30,000 square foot state of the art office building in Hauppauge, New York. First year that LIAAC was the recipient agency of the Chef's Secrets fundraiser. During its annual meeting in January, the World Economic Forum approved a set of new priorities, including one, with a focus on addressing HIV/AIDS in Africa and other hard-hit regions. Also, on January 26th, the FDA grants tentative approval to a generic co-packaged antiretroviral drug regimen for use under the *United States President's Emergency Plan for AIDS Relief* (PEPFAR). May 19th is the first annual National Asian and Pacific Islander HIV/AIDS Awareness Day in the U.S.

2006

LIAAC's first non-HIV/AIDS specific grant awarded from the *New York State Department of Health Hunger Prevention Nutrition Assistance Program* (HPNAP) allowed us to establish the Pantry on Wheels and bring pantry bags to the food insecure living in some of Long Island's most disenfranchised communities. Then came a revised mission statement to reflect that non-HIV related services are an integral part of LIAAC. LIAAC received a grant from Federal Office of Minority Health, which includes BiasHELP and *Emergency Operations Center* (EOC) of Suffolk as key partners. LIAAC receives a grant from Substance Abuse and Mental Health Services Administration, Center for Substance Abuse Prevention to expand our testing capabilities as well as add Hepatitis C screening to their services.

LIAAC received funding from NY State Assembly to pilot a Crystal Meth prevention education program. LIAAC worked in partnership with LINCS (Community, Courses, and Resources for Adult Education on a NYS tobacco control grant and a Drug Free Communities grant. June 5th, marks 25 years since the first AIDS cases were reported. March 10 is the first annual National Women and Girls HIV/AIDS Awareness Day in the U.S. March 20th, was the first annual observance of National Native HIV/AIDS Awareness Day in the U.S. On September 22nd, the CDC released a revised HIV testing recommendation for healthcare settings, recommending routine HIV screening for all adults, aged 13-64, and yearly screening for those at high risk. On December 19th, the U.S. Congress reauthorizes the Ryan White CARE Act for the third time.

2007

LIAAC created a new logo for the organization, including the phrase: "Solving the Challenges of HIV" Re-named organizational newsletter from the LIAAC Voice to the LIAAC Challenge. LIAAC is awarded the Ryan White Title I Outreach Grant to design and execute mass media HIV/AIDS awareness campaign on Long Island to reach out-of-care individuals. The "I Get Care" Hotline was established. In June, the Rwandan Government hosts the International HIV/AIDS implementers meeting. Over 1,500 delegates shared lessons on HIV prevention, treatment and care. Co-sponsors included WHO, UNAIDS, the United States PEPFAR, The Global Fund to Fight AIDS, tuberculosis, and malaria, UNICEF, the World Bank, and GNP+ (the *Global Network of People Living with HIV*). CDC reports over 565,000 people have died of AIDS in the U.S. since 1981.

2008

On August 6th, the CDC released new domestic HIV incidence estimates that were higher than previous estimates (56,300 new infections per year vs. 40,000). The new estimates did not represent an actual increase in the numbers of HIV infections but reflected a more accurate way of measuring new infections. A separate analysis suggested that the annual number of new infections was never as low as 40,000 and that it has been stable since the late 1990s. September 18th was the first observance of National HIV/AIDS and Aging Awareness Day. National Gay Men's HIV/AIDS Awareness Day is first recognized on September 27th.

2009

FOMH awarded LIAAC a grant for a collaborative project with EOC of Suffolk and BiasHELP, Inc. This project, *Health Improvements for Re-entering Ex-offend-*

ers (H.I.R.E.) was a three-pronged approach to provide health, economic and recidivism prevention services to individuals returning to Long Island from federal or state incarceration who were either currently infected with HIV/AIDS or at high risk for infection. Newly elected President Barack Obama calls for the development of the first National HIV/AIDS Strategy for the United States. In February, the District of Columbia Health Department's HIV/AIDS, Hepatitis, *Sexually Transmitted Diseases* (STD's), and Tuberculosis (TB) Administration reports that Washington, DC had a higher rate of HIV, a 3% prevalence over that in West Africa, enough to describe it as a "severe and generalized epidemic.". June 8th marked the first annual recognition of Caribbean American HIV/AIDS Awareness Day. On October 6th, the U.S. FDA, in association with the PEPFAR program, approved the 100th antiretroviral drug. On October 30, President Obama announces that his administration will officially lift the HIV travel and immigration ban in January 2010 by removing the final regulatory barriers for entry. The lifting of the travel ban occurred in conjunction with the announcement that the International AIDS Conference will return to the United States for the first time in more than 20 years. The conference was held in Washington, DC, in 2012.

2010

LIAAC is the only agency on Long Island to be directly funded by the CDC, through a five-year cooperative agreement. This agreement enabled LIAAC to continue to conduct HIV Counseling, rapid Testing and Referral as well as introduce Safety Counts, an evidence-based intervention, to at-risk Long Islanders. LIAAC is awarded a grant from the Substance Abuse and Mental Health Services Administration, Center for Substance Abuse Prevention to implement "The Seasoned Adults Project." This project added to their comprehensive services, blended substance abuse and HIV, hepatitis C and STD prevention, referral and testing services to at-risk ethnic and/or racial minority older adults (50 and older), who reside in and/or frequent Long Island communities that were burdened with a disproportionate incidence/prevalence of HIV/AIDS and Substance Abuse.

On January 4th, the U.S. Government officially lifted the HIV travel and immigration ban. On March 23rd, President Obama signs the *Patient Protection and Affordable Care Act* (PPACA), which expanded access to care and prevention for all Americans but offered special protections for those living with chronic illnesses, like HIV, that made it difficult for them to access or afford healthcare. On July 13th, the Obama Administration released the first comprehensive National HIV/AIDS Strategy for the United States. AIDS Action merged with the National AIDS Fund to form AIDS United.

2011

LIAAC enters into a sole source agreement with the NYSDOH, Bureau of HIV/AIDS Epidemiology to collaborate on the *National HIV Behavioral Surveillance* (NHBS) research project, a joint effort by the NYSDOH, *Bureau of HIV/AIDS Epidemiology* (BHAE) and the CDC. This research was a part of a multi-state, personal interview survey of people at high risk for HIV. The study sought to collect comprehensive information about sexual and drug-use risk behaviors, HIV testing histories and exposure to and use of HIV prevention services among those at the highest risk of infection. In recognition of its dedication and commitment for the betterment of the Long Island community, LIAAC is awarded the Bank of America Elena M. Perez Memorial Grant. Public debate began on whether the longstanding ban on transplants of HIV-infected organs should be dropped. The HHS launched the 12 Cities Project, an HHS-wide project that supported and accelerated comprehensive HIV/AIDS planning and cross-agency response in the 12 U.S. jurisdictions that bear the highest AIDS burden in the country.

AIDS activist and award-winning actress Elizabeth Taylor died on March 23rd. One of the first celebrities to advocate on behalf of people living with HIV and AIDS, Taylor was the founding national chairman of *The American Foundation for Aids Research* (amfAR) a non-profit organization that supported AIDS research, HIV prevention, treatment education, and advocates for AIDS-related public policy. On June 8th, HHS Secretary Sebelius hosted "Commemorating 30 Years of Leadership in the Fight Against HIV/AIDS".

2012

March 13th Researchers from the University of New South Wales in Australia find that people living with HIV who are taking antiretroviral therapy have an increased risk of cardiovascular disease .The U.S. Department of Health and Human Services issues new HIV treatment guidelines recommending treatment for all HIV-infected adults and adolescents, regardless of CD4 count or viral load on March 27th.

July 1st, the Kaiser Family Foundation and the *Washington Post* release a joint survey of the American public's attitudes, awareness, and experiences related to HIV and AIDS. The survey finds that roughly a quarter of Americans do *not* know that HIV cannot be transmitted by sharing a drinking glass—almost exactly the same share as in 1987.

On July 3rd, the FDA approves the first at-home HIV test that will let users learn their HIV status right away.

July 16th, The FDA approves the use of Truvada® for pre-exposure prophylaxis (PrEP). Adults who do not have HIV, but who are at risk for infection, can now take this medication to reduce their risk of getting the virus through sexual activity.

July 22nd-27th, the XIX International AIDS Conference (AIDS 2012) is held in Washington, DC; the first time since 1990 that the conference has been held in the United States. Conference organizers had refused to convene the event in the U.S. until the Federal government lifted the ban on HIV-positive travelers entering the country.

During AIDS 2012, the AIDS Memorial Quilt is displayed in its entirety in Washington, DC, for the first time since 1996. Volunteers have to rotate nearly

50,000 panels to ensure that the entire work is displayed. Microsoft Research, the University of Southern California, the NAMES Project Foundation, and a handful of other institutions collaborate to create a zoomable "map" of the Quilt. The U.S. President's Emergency Plan for AIDS Relief (PEPFAR) celebrates its 10th anniversary.

March 4th, NIH-funded scientists announce the first well-documented case of an HIV-infected child, designated as "the Mississippi Baby," who appears to have been functionally cured of HIV infection (i.e., no detectable levels of virus or signs of disease, even without antiretroviral therapy.

2013

June 2nd, the New York Times runs two articles which focus on middle-aged people living with HIV: The Faces of H.I.V. in New York in 2013 and 'People Think It's Over': Spared Death, Aging People With H.I.V. Struggle to Live . The National Minority AIDS Council (NMAC) releases RISE Proud: Combating HIV Among Black Gay and Bisexual Men (PDF 1.4 MB), an action plan to mitigate the impact of HIV on black gay and bisexual men on June 5th. On June 18th, Secretary of State John Kerry announces that, thanks to direct PEP-

FAR support, more than 1 million infants have been born HIV-free since 2003.

Then, on July 3rd, Researchers report that two HIV-positive patients in Boston who had bone-marrow transplants for blood cancers have apparently been virus-free for weeks since their antiretroviral drugs were stopped.

July 13th, President Obama issues an Executive Order directing Federal agencies to prioritize supporting the HIV care continuum as a means of implementing the National HIV/AIDS Strategy. The HIV Care Continuum Initiative aims to accelerate efforts to improve the percentage of people living with HIV who move from testing to treatment and ultimately, to viral suppression.

October, The National Latino AIDS Action Network (NLAAN), a diverse coalition of community-based organizations, national organizations, state and local health departments, researchers and concerned individuals, publishes the National Latino/Hispanic HIV/AIDS Action Agenda (PDF 4.1 MB) to raise awareness, identify priorities, and issue specific recommendations to address the impact of the epidemic in Hispanic/Latino communities.

November 21th, President Obama signs the *HIV Organ Policy Equity* (HOPE) Act, which will allow people living with HIV to receive organs from other infected donors. The HOPE Act has the potential to save the lives of about 1,000 HIV-infected patients with liver and kidney failure annually.

December 5th, Nelson Mandela—South African anti-apartheid leader, political prisoner, and national President from 1994 to 1999—dies at the age of 95. After his son, Makgatho, died of AIDS-related causes in 2005, Mandela spent the remainder of his post presidential career working to address the AIDS epidemic in South Africa, which is home to the largest number of people living with HIV (~6.8 million) in the world.

At the end of 2012, UNAIDS estimates that, worldwide, 2.3 million people were newly infected with HIV during the year, and 1.6 million people died of AIDS. Approximately 35.3 million people around the world are now living with HIV, including more than 1.2 million Americans.

UNAIDS also announces that new HIV infections have dropped more than 50% in 25 low- and middle-income countries, and the number of people getting antiretroviral treatment has increased 63% in the past two years.

2014

On June 29th, 2014 Governor Cuomo, the 56th New York Governor announced a three-point plan to reduce HIV infections from 3000 -750 by the year 2020. The plan includes: (1) Identifying HIV undiagnosed persons and linking them to health care; (2) Linking and retaining HIV diagnosed persons in health care and maintaining antiretroviral therapy for viral load suppression in order to remain healthy and prevent transmission; (3) Facilitate access to *Pre-Exposure Prophylaxis* (PrEP) for high-risk negative persons. To implement the "bending the curve" three-point plan, LIAAC had worked closely with local Departments of Health and legislators to develop prevention education community programs; and had signed memorandums of agreements and service provider agreements with various primary care, pharmaceutical, mental health and substance abuse treatment organizations. In addition, they have retrained their staff in linkage/retention in care and patient navigation strategies; also updated public health information for their hotline, social media platforms and community resource directory for accessing infectious disease doctors, PrEP and other prevention supportive services in Suffolk and Nassau Counties.

September 9th, The Pew Charitable Trust publishes Southern States Are Now Epicenter of HIV/AIDS in the U.S. October 9th, the CDC released a new report that found gaps in care and treatment among Latinos diagnosed with HIV. On November 25th, the CDC announced that only 30% of Americans with HIV had the virus under control in 2011, and approximately two-thirds of those whose virus was out of control had been diagnosed but were no longer under care.

December 23rd, the FDA announced it will recommend changing the blood donor deferral guidelines for men who have sex with men from permanent deferral to one year since the last sexual contact. In 1983, the agency imposed a lifetime ban on donating blood for all men who have ever had sex with another man.

2015

January 8th, a review of multiple studies of South African women indicated that using Depo Provera, an injectable contraceptive, may increase women's chances of contracting HIV by 40 percent. February 5th, HHS announced the launch of a new, 4-year demonstration project to address HIV disparities among *Men-who-have sex-with Men* (MSM) of color. The cross-agency project, "Developing Comprehensive Models of HIV Prevention and Care Services for MSM of Color," supported community-based models for HIV prevention and treatment.

February 23rd, the CDC's annual HIV Surveillance Report indicated that HIV diagnosis rates in the U.S. remained stable between 2009-2013, but men who have sex with men, young adults, racial/ethnic minorities, and individuals living in the South continued to bear a disproportionate burden of HIV. On that same day, the CDC announced that more than 90% of new HIV infections in the United States could be prevented by diagnosing people living with HIV and ensured they would receive prompt, ongoing care and treatment.

On February 25th, Indiana state health officials announced an HIV outbreak linked to injection drug use in the southeastern portion of the state. By the end of the year, Indiana confirmed 184 new cases of HIV linked to the outbreak. On April 15th, NIH launched a large, multi-center, international clinical trial to study heart disease in people living with HIV, who statistics proved are twice as likely as HIV-negative individuals to have heart attacks and other forms of cardiovascular disease.

On May 8th, the HHS announced that it would amend the Federal rules covering organ transplants to allow the recovery of transplantable organs from

HIV-positive donors. The new regulations provided a framework for clinical studies on transplanting organs from HIV-positive donors to HIV-positive recipients.

On May 27th, results from the *Strategic Timing of AntiRetroviral Treatment* (START) study indicated that HIV-positive individuals who start taking antiretroviral drugs before their CD4+ cell counts decrease, have a considerably lower risk of developing AIDS or other serious illnesses. Subsequent data released showed that early therapy for people living with HIV also prevented the onset of cancer, cardiovascular disease, and other non-AIDS-related diseases.

On June 30th, WHO certified that Cuba was the first nation to eliminate mother-to-child transmission of both HIV and syphilis. July 14th, UNAIDS announced that the targets for Millennium Development Goal #6, halting and reversing the spread of HIV had been achieved and exceeded nine months ahead of the schedule set in 2000. July 20th, researchers reported that antiretroviral therapy was highly effective at preventing sexual transmission of HIV from a person living with HIV to an uninfected heterosexual partner, when the HIV-positive partner is virally suppressed. The finding comes from the decade-long HPTN 052 clinical trial.

On July 23rd, the FDA approved the first diagnostic test that differentiated between different types of HIV infections (HIV-1 and HIV-2). The test also differentiated between acute and established HIV infections. July 30th, the White House launched the National HIV/AIDS Strategy: The updated Strategy retained the vision and goals of the original, but reflected scientific advances, transformations in healthcare access as a result of the ACA and a renewed emphasis on key populations, geographic areas, and practices necessary to end the domestic HIV epidemic.

On September 18th, the U.S. Department of *Housing and Urban Development* (HUD) and Justice announced they would collaborate on a demonstration project to provide housing assistance and supportive services to low-income persons living with HIV/AIDS who are victims of sexual assault, domestic violence, dating violence, or stalking. September 26th, at a United Nations summit on the Sustainable Development Goals, the United States announced new PEPFAR prevention and treatment targets for 2016–2017. By the end of 2017, the U.S. committed sufficient resources to support antiretroviral therapy for 12.9 million people and reduced HIV incidence by 40% among adolescent girls and young women within the highest burdened areas of 10 sub-Saharan African countries.

On September 30th, WHO announced new treatment recommendations that called for all people living with HIV to begin antiretroviral therapy as possible after diagnosis. WHO also recommended daily oral PrEP as an additional prevention choice for those at substantial risk for contracting HIV. WHO estimated the new policy could help avert more than 21 million deaths and 28 million new infections by 2030.

October 20th, *Greater Than AIDS* launched a new campaign, *Empowered: Women, HIV and Intimate Partner Violence,* to bring more attention to issues of relationship violence and provided resources for women who may be at risk of, or dealing with, abuse and HIV. November 17th, actor Charlie Sheen announced his HIV positive status in a nationally televised interview. Significant public conversation about HIV followed his disclosure. Earlier in the year, rapper, performance artist, and poet Mykki Blanco took to Facebook to disclose his HIV status, and former child TV star Danny Pintauro told Oprah that he is living with HIV.

November 24th, UNAIDS released its 2015 World AIDS Day report which found that 15.8 million people were accessing antiretroviral treatment as of June 2015, now more than doubling the number of people who were on treatment in 2010. November 30th, amfAR, announced its plan to establish the amfAR Institute for HIV Cure Research at the University of California, San Francisco. As the cornerstone of amfAR's $100 million investment in cure research, the Institute would work to develop the scientific basis for an HIV cure by the end of 2020.

December 1st, the White House released a Federal Action Plan to accompany the updated National HIV/AIDS Strategy. The plan was developed by 10 Federal agencies and the Equal Employment Opportunity Commission (EEOC) and contained 170 action items that the agencies would undertake to achieve the goals of the Strategy.

December 6th, the CDC announced that annual HIV diagnoses in the U.S. fell by 19% from 2005 to 2014. There were steep declines among heterosexuals, IV drug users, and African Americans (especially black women), but trends for gay/bisexual men varied by race/ethnicity. Dragonesses among white gay/bisexual men had decreased by 18%, but they continued to rise among Latino gay/bisexual men and were up 24%. Diagnoses among black gay/bisexual men also increased 22%, but the increase has since leveled off since 2010.

December 19th, partly in response to the HIV outbreak in Indiana, which is linked to people injecting drugs, Congress lifts restrictions that prevented states and localities from spending Federal funds for needle exchange programs. December 21st, the FDA announced it would lift the 30-year-old ban on all blood donations by men who have sex with men and institute a policy that allows them to donate blood if they have not had sexual contact with another man in the previous 12 months.

2016

On January 19th 2016, the CDC reported that only 1 in 5 sexually active high school students had been tested for HIV. An estimated 50% of young Americans who are living with HIV do not know they are infected.

January 28th, researchers announced that an international study of over 1,900 patients with HIV who failed to respond to the antiretroviral drug *tenofovir*, a key HIV treatment medication indicates that HIV resistance to the medication had become increasingly common. February 25th, during the annual *Conference on Retroviruses and Opportunistic Infections* (CROI), researchers reported that a man taking the HIV-prevention pill *Truvada* had contracted HIV, marking the first reported infection of someone regularly taking the drug.

March 3rd, the White House Office of National AIDS Policy, the NIH Office of AIDS Research, and the National Institute of Mental Health cohost a meeting to address the issue of HIV stigma: Translating Research to Action: Reducing HIV Stigma to Optimize HIV Outcomes. Participants included researchers, policymakers, legal scholars, faith leaders, advocates, and people living with HIV.

March 3rd, Pharmacy researchers reported finding that women need daily doses of the antiviral medication Truvada to prevent HIV infection, while men only need two doses per week due to differences in the way the drug accumulates in vaginal, cervical and rectal tissue. March 29th, HHS released new guidance for state, local, tribal, and territorial health departments that would allow them to request permission to use federal funds to SSPs. The funds can now be used to support a comprehensive set of services, but they cannot be used to purchase sterile needles or syringes for illegal drug injection.

May 24th, the NOIH and partners announced they will launch a large HIV vaccine trial in South Africa in November 2016, pending regulatory approval. This represented the first time since 2009 that the scientific community has embarked on an HIV vaccine clinical trial of this size. June 8th-10th, the UN held its 2016 High-Level Meeting on Ending AIDS . UN member states pledge to end the AIDS epidemic by 2030, but the meeting is marked by controversy after more than 50 nations block the participation of groups representing LGBT people from the meeting. The final resolution barely mentions those most at risk for contracting HIV/AIDS: men who have sex with men, sex workers, transgender people and people who inject drugs.

2017

January 16th, the CDC reports that more people were diagnosed with AIDS in 1985 than in all earlier years combined. The 1985 figures show an 89% increase in new AIDS cases compared with 1984. Of all AIDS cases to date, 51% of adults and 59% of children have died. The new report shows that, on average, AIDS patients die about 15 months after the disease is diagnosed. Public health experts predict twice as many new AIDS cases in 1986.

On May 1st, The International Committee on the Taxonomy of Viruses announces that the virus that causes

AIDS will officially be known as "Human Immunodeficiency Virus" (HIV).

July 18th, at the *National Conference on AIDS in the Black Community* in Washington, DC, a group of minority leaders meets with the U.S. Surgeon General, Dr. C. Everett Koop, to discuss concerns about HIV/AIDS in communities of color. This meeting marks the unofficial founding of the National Minority AIDS Council.

October, the Robert Wood Johnson Foundation creates the *AIDS Health Services Program*, providing $17.2 million in funding for patient-care demonstration projects in 11 cities. The goal is to replicate the San Francisco Model of Care nationwide—but with an emphasis on tailoring programs to meet the needs in local contexts.

Later in October, the U.S. Health Resources and Services Administration (HRSA) begins its AIDS Service Demonstration Grants program—the agency's first AIDS-specific health initiative. In the program's first year, HRSA makes $15.3 million available to four of the country's hardest-hit cities: New York, San Francisco, Los Angeles, and Miami.

October 22nd, the Surgeon General issues the *Surgeon General's Report on AIDS*. The report makes it clear that HIV cannot be spread casually and calls for: a nationwide education campaign (including early sex education in schools); increased use of condoms; and voluntary HIV testing.

October 24th, the CDC reports that AIDS cases are disproportionately affecting African Americans and Latinos. This is particularly true for African American and Latinx children, who make up 90% of perinatally acquired AIDS cases.

October 29th, the Institute of Medicine (IOM), the principal health unit of the National Academy of Sciences, issues a report, *Confronting AIDS: Directions for Public Health, Health Care, and Research*. The report calls for a "massive media, educational and public health campaign to curb the spread of the HIV infection," as well as for the creation of a National Commission on AIDS. The IOM estimates that the effort will require a $2 billion investment in research and patient care by the end of the decade.

2018

January 15th, Dr. Mathilde Krim dies at age 91. Dr. Krim, a geneticist and virologist who turned from studying cancer to studying AIDS, started the AIDS Medical Foundation in 1983, and then became the founding chairwoman of the Foundation for AIDS Research (amfAR) in 1985. She raised hundreds of millions of dollars for AIDS research, prevention, treatment, and advocacy. In announcing her passing, the *New York Times* calls her "America's foremost warrior in the battle against superstitions, fears and prejudices that have stigmatized many people with AIDS ."

January 24th, the National Institutes of Health launches a large international study to compare the safety and efficacy of antiretroviral treatment regimens for pregnant women living with HIV and their infants. It will provide data on the use of newer HIV medications during pregnancy, helping to ensure that women living with HIV and their infants receive the best available treatments.

On January 28th, PEPFAR (the President's Emergency Plan for AIDS Relief) celebrates its 15th anniversary. When PEPFAR began in 2003, only 50,000 people in Africa were on lifesaving HIV treatment. PEPFAR now supports over 14 million people on treatment globally.

April 16th, after a former boyfriend threatens to blackmail her over her HIV status, Austrian singer and Eurovision winner Conchita tells her fans that she is HIV-positive . In a press statement, she notes that she has been in treatment and virally suppressed for many years and says 'I hope to show courage and take another step against the stigmatization of people with HIV."

May 3rd, an international research team finds that early antiretroviral therapy (ART) is key to avoiding brain atrophy for people living with HIV . Using magnetic resonance imaging (MRI) data, researchers found that the longer people living with HIV went without treatment, the greater the atrophy in several brain regions. Once patients began ART, the atrophy stopped and some brain volume and was restored—demonstrating the importance of early screening and ART initiation.

After one month, on June 11th, In the first study to focus specifically on the effect of sustained viral suppression on overall cancer risk, researchers find that early, sustained antiretroviral therapy resulting in long-term viral suppression helps to prevent AIDS-defining cancers and—to a lesser degree—other cancers for people living with HIV. But the long-term study (1999-2015), which followed nearly 150,000 veterans, also found that patients with long-term viral suppression still had excess cancer risk compared to HIV-negative patients.

June 28th, in a Northwestern University study, "Keep It Up!", a novel online HIV-prevention program that targets young men who have sex with men (MSM), between the ages of 18-29, reduces sexually transmitted infections by 40%. The program, which offers video clips, soap operas, and interactive games is the first online HIV-prevention program to show effects on a biological outcome.

July 18th, a global analysis finds that people living with HIV are twice as likely as their HIV-negative counterparts to suffer from heart disease . Based on a review of studies with almost 800,000 people from 153 countries, an international team of experts finds that HIV-associated cardiovascular disease has more than tripled in the past 20 years as more people live longer with the virus.

August 1st, researchers at Los Alamos National Laboratory demonstrate that computer simulations can accurately predict the transmission of HIV across populations . The simulations are consistent with 840,000 actual HIV DNA sequences contained in a global public HIV database. The simulations could allow state health departments to track the spread of HIV and provide a powerful new tool to help prevent new HIV infections.

September 7th, The Office of HIV/AIDS and Infectious Disease Policy, in the U.S. Department of Health and Human Services (HHS), hosts the first in a series of listening sessions to begin updating the National HIV/AIDS Strategy and the National Viral Hepatitis Action Plan. The session is held as part of activities at the U.S. Conference on AIDS in Orlando, Florida, and is attended by HIV community leaders, frontline workers, individuals living with and at risk for infection, and other stakeholders from across the nation.

September 28th, a study of MSM in Thailand finds that having a sexually transmitted infection does not affect the ability of people living with HIV to achieve and maintain an undetectable viral load . The results confirm the generalizability of the "Undetectable = Untransmittable" (U=U) message.

A bit later in October, a new study reports that targeted, high-coverage roll-out of pre-exposure prophylaxis (PrEP) was associated with a 25% reduction in new HIV diagnoses in one year . The study followed 3,700 MSM in New South Wales, Australia, who were taking PrEP with high levels of adherence. It is the first empirical study to test PrEP's population-level effectiveness.

November 20th, the U.S. Preventive Services Task Force, an independent, volunteer panel of national experts in prevention and evidence-based medicine, issues a draft recommendation that clinicians should offer PrEP to individuals at high risk for HIV infection. The Task Force gives its "A" recommendation—the strongest endorsement it can give—to PrEP, stating that, when taken as prescribed, PrEP is highly effective at preventing HIV among those at high risk, and concluding with "high certainty" that there is a substantial benefit to the target population.

December 1st, is the date marks the 30th anniversary of the observance of World AIDS Day.

(This timeline was retrieved from an official U.S. Government website managed by the U.S. Department of Health & Human Services (HHS) and supported by the *Secretary's Minority AIDS Initiative Fund* (SMAIF) and HIV.gov.

Transmission

There are several ways in which someone can become infected with HIV. These transmission routes are well defined. HIV infection can be transmitted through: Unprotected sexual intercourse with an infected partner; injection or transfusion of contaminated blood or blood products, through artificial insemination, skin grafts and organ transplants are also possible); sharing unsterilized injection equipment that has been previously used by someone who is infected; maternofetal transmission (during pregnancy, at birth, and through breast-feeding).

Sexual Intercourse

For sexual transmission of HIV, the risk of transmission is not constant for all sexual encounters. In understanding the risk of the sexual transmission of HIV, researchers often consider two broad categories:

1. the type of sex act, namely oral versus vaginal versus anal sex, and
2. biological and other factors, such as the level of virus in the HIV-positive partner or the presence of other sexually transmitted infections (STIs), that can decrease or increase risk.

Unprotected sexual intercourse is the most prevalent transmission route of HIV infection worldwide. Although receptive anal sex is estimated to produce the highest risk of infection, infection after a single insertive contact has also been described. The presence of other sexually transmitted diseases markedly increases the risk of becoming infected with HIV. Unprotected sexual intercourse is the most important transmission route of HIV infection worldwide. Although receptive anal sex is estimated to produce the highest risk of infection, infection after a single insertive contact has also been described. The presence of other sexually transmitted diseases markedly increases the risk of becoming infected with HIV.

The lower the viral load, the less infectious the patient. A prospective study of 415 HIV-discordant couples in Uganda showed that of 90 new infections occurring over a period of up to 30 months, none was from an infected partner with a viral load below 1,500 copies/ml. The risk of infection increased with every log of viral load by a factor of 2.45. It should be noted that the levels of viral load in blood and other body fluids do not always correlate with one another. Thus, individual risk remains difficult to estimate.

The higher the viral load, the more infectious the patient. This is especially true for patients during acute HIV infection. During acute HIV-1 infection, the virus replicates extensively in the absence of any detectable adaptive immune response reaching levels of over 100 million copies of HIV-1 RNA/ml.

Intravenous Drug Use

Injection drug use-related HIV infection accounts for a substantial and growing fraction of the total cases of HIV in the United States. Injection drug use has spread HIV rapidly across the U.S and also in parts of Europe and Asia. Risk factors for HIV infection among injection drug users (IDUs) include demographic characteristics and practices that increase sexual transmission and parenteral exposure to infected blood. This will describe the epidemiology, prevalence, and incidence of HIV infection among IDUs in the United States and abroad, and preventive interventions, including addiction treatment, risk-reduction education, the use of disinfectants, and the provision of sterile injection equipment.

Sharing unsterilized injection equipment that has been previously used by someone who is infected is another common route of HIV transmission in many countries with a high prevalence of intravenous drug users. In my personal case, I believe this was how I contracted the virus. One may never know exactly how or pin it down to one sexual encounter. In contrast to the accidental needle stick injury, the risk of transmission through sharing injection equipment is far higher.

Transmission of HIV among IDUs occurs primarily through HIV-infected blood contamination of injection paraphernalia, which is re-used by an uninfected IDU. Behaviors that increase the likelihood, frequency, and magnitude of exposure to infected blood increase the risk of infection. Among IDUs, several demographic and behavioral characteristics are associated with greater risk of acquiring HIV. Residence in or near an area of high prevalence is a powerful risk factor, both domestically as just described and worldwide.

Within the United States, other very consistent independent predictors of HIV seroprevalence among IDUs include: minority race or ethnicity, low income, male gender, and a diagnosis of antisocial personality disorder. African-American and Hispanic IDUs have significantly higher seroprevalence than of Caucasian, non-Hispanic IDUs in New York, Connecticut, and San Francisco.

Gender differences in HIV infection vary geographically, from New York, where seroprevalence is 13% greater among male than among female IDUs, to San Francisco, where the seroprevalence among men and women IDUs is identical. Antisocial personality disorder (APD), which is prevalent in 40% of IDUs, as compared with 3% of the general population, is associated with more frequent injection, more frequent needle sharing with a greater number of partners, and greater use of alcohol and cocaine.

Until recently, no biological differences in susceptibility to acquiring HIV had been demonstrated to explain the different rates of infection among different demographic, racial, ethnic, and gender groupings. Recent reports describe a nucleotide deletion with the beta-chemokine receptor (CCR5) gene that is strongly associated with remaining uninfected despite frequent sexual exposure to HIV. This allele was found in 8% of white gay men enrolled at the Chicago site of the Multicenter AIDS Cohort Study, but in no participants of African or Asian descent. It is likely that other, as yet undiscovered genetic correlates of race, ethnicity, and gender that confer resistance or susceptibility will explain some of the variability in infection rates.

Maternofetal

In the absence of any intervention it is estimated 15-30% of mothers with HIV infection will transmit the infection during pregnancy and delivery. In approximately 75% of these cases, HIV is transmitted during late pregnancy or during delivery. About 10% of vertical HIV infections occur before the third trimester, and 10-15% are caused by breastfeeding. In Western countries, perinatal (vertical) HIV infection has become rare since the introduction of antiretroviral transmission prophylaxis and elective caesarean section.

Mother-to-child transmission of human immune deficiency virus HIV is a multifactorial event highly associated with advanced maternal HIV disease and obstetric incidents that takes place during parturition. Thus, various approaches to prevention may be beneficial. Although the time and the route of maternofetal HIV transmission are still to this day, are not sufficiently clear, much speaks in favor of a late HIV transmission, most probably taking place during parturition or the phase before the delivery. The fetus is remarkably protected by the placenta and the intact fetal membranes against many viral infections during gestation. These conditions change at parturition and the chance for a transition of HIV-infected carrier cells or virus into the fetal compartment increases. Proinflammatory cytokines secreted at the maternofetal interface accumulate in amniotic fluid and may chemoattract and stimulate potentially HIV-infected immunocytes. After rupture of membranes, maternal cells of the decidua are directly exposed to the amniotic fluid. Aside from the contamination of the fetal skin at vaginal delivery as a debatable route of infection, blood-to-blood contacts and the fetal swallowing of contaminated amniotic fluid may be the major path of fetal HIV infection.

For the fetal prophylaxis of an intrauterine infection, the application of zidovudine is recommended. However, caesarian section before the onset of labor leads also to a diminution of the transmission rate. As the transmission seems to have both systemic and local causes, it makes sense to combine different intervention strategies. Whether a combination of zidovudine and elective caesarean section can lower the transmission risk further has to be evaluated.

Injection or Transfusion of Contaminated Blood Products

In most Western countries, administration or transfusion of HIV-contaminated blood, or blood products has become a rare event. With current testing methods, the risk of acquiring HIV from a unit of transfused blood is about 1: 1,000,000, however, while Western European countries, and the United States, Australia, Canada, and Japan have strict and mandatory screening of donated blood for HIV.

HIV cannot be transmitted as easily as the influenza virus, as compared to other viral diseases, and the prevention of HIV infection is therefore easier. In rich countries, individuals who do not want to be infected with HIV may protect themselves and avoid HIV infection. The same people will not be able to avoid the influenza virus of the next pandemic. Outside these havens of material well-being, things have not changed since the early years of the HIV epidemic 35 years ago. Many people live in a world where no medical progress seems to have been made. This is a shameful situation, and hopefully future generations will more medical research will be more promising.

Transmission of HIV through transfusion of contaminated blood components was documented in the United States in 1982. Since then, the risk for transfusion-transmitted HIV infection has been almost eliminated by the use of questionnaires to exclude donors at higher risk for HIV infection and the use of highly sensitive laboratory screening tests to identify infected blood donations. The risk for acquiring HIV infection through blood transfusion today is estimated conservatively to be one in 1.5 million, based on 2007-2008 data. This report describes the first U.S. case of transfusion-transmitted HIV infection reported to CDC since

2002. A blood center in Missouri discovered that blood components from a donation in November 2008 tested positive for HIV infection.

A lookback investigation determined that this donor had last donated in June 2008, at which time he incorrectly reported no HIV risk factors and his donation tested negative for the presence of HIV. One of the two recipients of blood components from this donation, a patient undergoing kidney transplantation, was found to be HIV infected, and an investigation determined that the patient's infection was acquired from the donor's blood products. Even though similar transmissions are rare, health-care providers should consider the possibility of transfusion-transmitted HIV in HIV-infected transfusion recipients with no other risk factors.

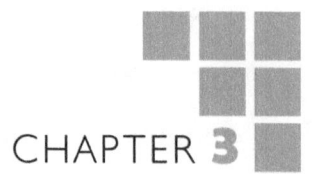

CHAPTER 3

NATURAL HISTORY

THE ACUTE viral syndrome of primary HIV infection, that was initially named HTLV-III, (*Human T-Lymphotropic Virus Type III*) LAV (*Lymphadenopathy Associated Virus*) ARV (*AIDS Associated Retrovirus*).

(which is the time period from initial infection with HIV to the development of an antibody response) shows symptoms that often resemble those of *mononucleosis*. These appear within days to weeks following exposure to HIV. However, these clinical signs and symptoms may not occur in all patients. During acute HIV infection, there is usually a high plasma viremia and frequently a marked decrease in *CD4+* T-cells. The CD4+ T-cell count later increases again, normally to levels inferior to the pre-infection values. After the acute infection, equilibrium between viral replication and the host immune response is usually reached, and many infected individuals may have no clinical manifestations of HIV infection for several years, even in the absence of antiretroviral treatment, this period of latency may last 8-10 years or more.

However, the term "latency period" can be a bit misleading, given the incredibly high turnover of the virus and the relentless daily destruction of CD4+ T-cells. At the end of the latency period, a number of symptoms or illnesses may appear which do not fulfill the definition of AIDS. These include slight immunological, dermatological, hematological and neurological signs.

HIV-1 Transmission Event

Acute HIV-1 infection presents in 40-90% of cases as a transient symptomatic illness, associated with high levels of HIV-1 replication and an expansive virus-specific immune response. With 14,000 new cases per day worldwide, it is an important differential diagnosis in cases of fever of unknown origin, maculopapular rash and lymphadenopathy. The diagnosis of acute infection is missed in the majority of cases, as other viral illnesses are often assumed to be the cause of the symptoms, and there are no HIV-1-specific antibodies detectable at this early stage of infection. The diagnosis therefore requires a high degree of clinical suspicion, based on clinical symptoms and history of exposure, in addition to specific laboratory tests (detection of HIV-1 RNA or p24 antigen and negative HIV-1 antibodies) confirming the diagnosis. An accurate early diagnosis of acute HIV-1 infection is important, as infection of sexual partners can be prevented, and patients may benefit from therapy at this early stage of infection.

The risk of infection associated with different exposure routes varies, but no matter what the transmission route, the timing of the appearance of viral and host markers of infection is uniform and follows an orderly pattern. Immediately after exposure and transmission, as HIV-1 is replicating in the mucosa, submucosa, and draining lymphoreticular tissues the virus cannot be detected in plasma; this so-called eclipse phase lasts 7 to 21 days. Once HIV-1 RNA reaches a concentration of 1 to 5 copies per milliliter in plasma, the virus can be detected with the use of sensitive qualitative methods of nucleic acid amplification; at concentrations of 50 copies per milliliter, HIV-1 can be detected by means of quantitative clinical assays used to monitor viral load.

The stages that define acute and early HIV-1 infection are characterized by the sequential appearance of viral markers and antibodies in the blood. More sensitive, fourth-generation tests, which detect both antigens and antibodies, shrink the virus-positive–antibody-negative window by about five days. Testing for viral RNA in plasma closes this gap by an additional seven days.

During acute HIV-1 infection, the virus replicates extensively in the absence of any detectable adaptive immune response, reaching levels of over 100 million copies HIV-1 RNA/ml. It is during this initial cycle of viral replication that important pathogenic processes are thought to occur. These include the seeding of virus to a range of tissue reservoirs and the destruction of CD4+ *T-lymphocytes*, in particular within the lymphoid tissues of the stomach. The very high levels of HIV-1 viremia are normally short-lived, indicating that the host is able to generate an immune response that controls viral replication. Over the following several weeks, viremia declines by several orders of magnitude before reaching a viral set point. This set point, following resolution of the acute infection, is a strong predictor of long-term disease progression rates.

Several factors can influence viral replication during acute infection and the establishment of a viral set point. These include the fitness of the infecting virus, host genetic factors and host immune responses. While antibodies against HIV-1 with neutralizing capacities are rarely detectable during primary HIV-1 infection, a number of studies have demonstrated a crucial role of HIV-1-specific cellular immune responses for the initial control of viral replication during this stage of infection. In addition to host immune responses, host genetic factors play an important role in both susceptibility and resistance to HIV-1 infection and speed of disease progression following infection. The most important of these is a deletion in the major co-receptor for entry of HIV-1 into CD4+ T-cells, a *chemokine* receptor called *CCR5*.

Signs and Symptoms

After an incubation period of a few days to a few weeks after exposure to HIV, most infected individuals present with an acute flu-like illness. Acute HIV-1 infection is a very heterogeneous syndrome and individuals presenting with more severe symptoms during acute infection and a longer duration of the acute infection syndrome tend to progress more rapidly to AIDS. The clinical symptoms of acute HIV-1 infection were first described in 1985 as an illness resembling infectious mononucleosis. The most common symptoms are fever, *maculopapular* rash, oral ulcers, *lymphadenopathy*, arthralgia, pharyngitis, malaise, weight loss, aseptic meningitis and myalgia.

In one study fever 80% and malaise 68% had the highest sensitivity for clinical diagnosis of acute HIV-1 infection, whereas loss of weight 86% and oral ulcers 85% had the highest specificity. In this study, the symptoms of fever and rash (especially in combination), followed by oral ulcers and pharyngitis had the highest positive predictive value for diagnosis of acute HIV-1 infection. In another study, fever, rash, myalgia, arthralgia and night sweats were the best predictors for acute HIV-1 infection.

The prevalence and incidence of HIV/AIDS vary considerably from continent to continent, from country to country and from region to region. Several countries in sub-Saharan Africa report infection rates of 30%, especially in urban areas. In other countries, HIV prevalence still remains low. However, low national prevalence rates can be misleading. They often disguise serious epidemics that are initially concentrated in certain localities or among specific population groups and that threaten to spill over into the wider population.

Diagnosis

The diagnosis of acute HIV-1 infection is based on the detection of HIV-1 replication in the absence of HIV-1 antibodies, which are not yet present at this early stage of infection. Different tests are available for diagnosis of acute HIV-1 infection. The most sensitive, accurate tests are based on detection of plasma HIV-1 RNA. During acute HIV-1 infection, there is frequently a marked decrease of *CD4+* T-cell count, which later increases again, but usually does not normalize to the initial levels. In contrast, the *CD8+* T-cell counts initially, which may result in a CD4/CD8 ratio of < 1. Infectious mononucleosis is the most important differential diagnosis. Hepatitis, influenza, toxoplasmosis, syphilis and side effects of medications should also be considered.

In summary, the most important step in the diagnosis of acute HIV-1 infection is to include it in the differential diagnosis. The clinical suspicion of an acute HIV-1 infection then merely requires performance of an HIV-1 antibody test and possibly repeated testing of HIV-1 viral load.

Treatment

Potential goals of antiretroviral therapy during acute HIV-1 infection are to shorten the symptomatic viral illness, reduce the number of infected cells, preserve HIV-1-specific immune responses, and lower the viral set point in the long term. Several studies in recent years have shown that treatment of acute HIV-1 infection allows long-term viral suppression, leads to preservation and even increase of HIV-1-specific T-helper cell responses and allows for the conservation of a very homogeneous virus population, but the clinical relevance of these findings is not known.

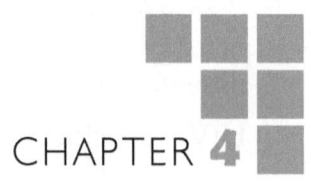

CHAPTER 4

HOW TO TEST

IT'S ALWAYS better to know!

Testing is the only way to know if you have HIV. It's normal to feel worried about HIV, but testing for HIV can help put your mind at ease and reduce the anxiety of not knowing. Whether your result is negative, or positive, it's always better to know so that you can move on with your life or start treatment if necessary. And remember, your result may not be what you expect.

A positive result means you can access treatment!

If you do have HIV, being diagnosed at an early stage means that you have a better chance of living a long and healthy life. This is because HIV attacks your immune system. If you're diagnosed early, you can start HIV treatment (antiretroviral drugs) earlier. This will lower the levels of HIV in your body, protect your immune system from damage, and stop you getting ill. With the right treatment and care, people living with HIV can expect to live as long as the average person, so it's important to take control of your health by getting a test.

Testing means you can keep your sexual partners healthy!

Testing for HIV regularly, and knowing your status, means that you can look after the sexual health of your partners too. If you're positive, you can prevent HIV from being transmitted to your partner by using condoms. Also, by starting and staying on antiretroviral treatment you will reduce the levels of HIV in your body, making it less likely you will pass HIV on. With effective antiretroviral treatment it's possible the level of virus in your body will go so low it becomes 'undetectable'. If this is confirmed by your healthcare professional, it means you can no longer pass on HIV through sex. If you find out you're positive, you can also encourage your partners to get tested!

Is HIV testing ever mandatory?

No, because choosing to take an HIV test can be hugely beneficial for yourself and your loved ones, the decision to test should be yours alone to make. However, some countries require you to get an HIV test in order to enter the country and in some countries, it is required for a marriage license. For further information about countries that have travel restriction, please see the Global Database on HIV travel. In addition, some insurance companies and employers such as the armed forces may require you to test for HIV. You should always seek advice from a healthcare professional first if you are unsure.

Awareness of one's HIV infection has gained enormous therapeutic relevance. Consequently, a shift in attitude towards HIV testing has taken place over the past decade, while an HIV test was previously often regarded as a threat to civil rights in the age of HAART, clinicians are to advise, if necessary, emphatically. Only those people who are aware of being infected can increase their life expectancy through HAART. Sometimes, an HIV test may be in the interest of a third person, e.g. testing of an index patient after a needle stick injury or the screening of pregnant women. Besides individual diagnostic use, HIV tests are used in large numbers in the screening of blood and organ donors and (often in an anonymous way) for epidemiological surveillance.

The diagnosis of an HIV infection is normally made indirectly, i.e. through the demonstration of virus-specific antibodies. These markers of a humeral immune response against the agent are found in virtually 100% of HIV-infected individuals. Their presence equals the diagnosis of chronic active HIV infection. Cases in which infected individuals persistently fail to have detectable antibodies against HIV are exceedingly rare and so far, play hardly any role in clinical practice. Besides indirect diagnosis based on detection of antibodies, a direct diagnosis of HIV infection is also possible: either through the demonstration of infectious virus (using cell culture - this is only possible in laboratories of at least biological safety level 3), of viral antigens (p24 antigen ELISA) or of viral nucleic acid (i.e. viral genome); the latter is also termed *nucleic acid testing* (*NAT*). Viral genome detection is nowadays most often used, as it does not require a high security laboratory, is more sensitive than antigen detection and allows quantification.

CHAPTER 5

CDC CLASSIFICATION

THE MOST widely accepted classification system of HIV infection, initially was published by the CDC in 1986, is was based on certain conditions associated with HIV infection. This classification system was intended for use in conducting public health surveillance and it has been a useful epidemiological tool for many years. In 1993, the CDC classification was revised and since then, the clinical definition of AIDS has been expanded in the USA (not in Europe) to include HIV-infected patients with a CD4+T-cell count of less than 200 cells/µl or less than 14% of all lymphocytes, even in the absence of the listed conditions. Persons infected with the etiologic retrovirus of acquired immunodeficiency syndrome AIDS may present a variety of manifestations, ranging from asymptomatic infection to severe immunodeficiency and life-threatening secondary infectious diseases or cancers. The rapid growth of knowledge about (HTLV-III/LAV) has resulted in an increasing need for a system of classifying patients within this spectrum of clinical and laboratory findings attributable to HTLV-III/LAV infection.

Various means are now being used to describe and assess patients with manifestations of HTLV-III/LAV infection and to describe the signs, symptoms, and laboratory findings. The surveillance definition of AIDS has proven to be extremely valuable and quite reliable for some epidemiologic studies and clinical assessment of patients with the more severe manifestations of disease However, more inclusive definitions and classifications of HTLV-III/LAV infection are needed for optimum patient care, health planning, and public health control strategies, as well as for epidemiologic studies and special surveys. A broadly applicable, easily understood classification system should also facilitate and clarify communication about this disease

CHAPTER 6

ANTIRETROVIRAL (ART) HISTORY

THERE IS not any field of medicine that has been through such dramatic developments as that of antiretroviral therapy. Very few other areas have been subject to such fast, and short-lived trends. Clinicians that have experienced the rapid developments in the last few years have been through many ups and downs. Following the hope in the early years, from 1987-1990, and the modest successes with monotherapy and the results of the Concorde Study plunged both patients and clinicians into a depression that was to last for several years. Azidothymidine, also called *Zidovudine*, (AZT), was introduced in March 1987 with great expectations, but did not seem to provide durable efficacy at least as a monotherapy and on early application. The same was true for the nucleoside analogs *ddC*, *ddI*, and *d4T*, introduced between

1991 and 1994. The lack of treatment options led to a debate that lasted for several years about which nucleoside analogs should be used, when, and what dose.

Many patients, who were infected up until the mid-80s, began to die. Hospices were established, as well as more and more support groups and ambulatory nursing services. One became accustomed to AIDS and its resulting death toll. There was, however, definite progress in the field of opportunistic infections, *cotrimoxazole, pentamidine, gancyclovir, foscarnet,* and *fluconazole* saved many patients lives, at least in the short-term.

Then, in September 1995, the results of the European-Australian DELTA Study and the American ACTG 175 Study attracted attention. It became apparent that two nucleoside analogs were more effective than monotherapy. Indeed, the differences made on the clinical endpoints, AIDS and death were highly significant. Both studies demonstrated that it was potentially of great importance of starting treatment immediately with two nucleoside analogs, as opposed to using the drugs successively.

This was by no means the final breakthrough, but by this time, the first studies with *protease inhibitors* (PIs), a completely new drug class, had been running for months. PIs had been designed using the knowledge of the molecular structure of HIV and protease in their clinical value was uncertain. Preliminary data, combined with rumours, were already circulating.

Patients and clinicians were waiting impatiently. In the fall of 1995, a fierce competition started up between Abbott, Roche and MSD. The licensing studies for the PIs, *ritonavir, saquinavir* and *indinavir*, were pursued with a great vigour. The monitors of these studies in the different companies lived for weeks in the clinical centers. Deep into the night, case report files had to be perfected and thousands of queries answered.

All these efforts led to a fast track approval, between December 1995 and March 1996, for all three PIs first saquinavir, followed by ritonavir and indinavir for the treatment of HIV. Many clinicians were not really aware of what was happening during these months. AIDS remained ever present. Patients were still dying, as only a relatively small number were participating in the PI trials and few were adequately treated according to current standards. And still several doubts remained. Hopes had been raised too many times before by alleged miracle cures. In January 1996, at the 5th Munich AIDS Conference, other topics were more important: palliative medicine, treatment of *cyto-*

megalovirus (CMV), wasting, and pain management; euthanasia was even a theme. The few contributions here and there on new beginnings produced no more than restrained optimism.

In February 1996, during the 3rd *Conference on Retroviruses and Opportunistic Infections* (CROI) in Washington, many caught their breath as Bill Cameron reported the first data from the ABT-247 Study during the late breaker session. The auditorium was absolutely silent, and electrified, listeners learned that the mere addition of ritonavir oral solution decreases the frequency of death and AIDS from 38% to 22%. These were sensational results in comparison to everything else that had been previously published.

Although some severely ill patients with AIDS managed to recover during these months, for many the combinations that were now at the beginning of 1996, widely used, came too late. Then in June 1996, the World AIDS Conference in Vancouver reported on the new AIDS cocktails and the strangely unscientific and ridiculous new expression *highly active antiretroviral therapy* (HAART) began to spread irreversibly. Clinicians were quite happy to become infected by this enthusiasm.

Meanwhile, David Ho, Time magazines Man of the Year in 1996, had clarified the hitherto completely misunderstood kinetics of HIV with his breakthrough trials. A year earlier, Ho had already initiated the slogan hit hard and early, and almost everyone was now taking him by his word. With the knowledge of the high turnover of the virus and the relentless daily destruction of CD4 cells, there was no consideration of a patient phase and no life without antiretroviral therapy. In many centers, almost every patient was treated. Within three years, from 1994-1997, the proportion of untreated patients in Europe decreased from 37% to 9%, whilst the proportion of HAART patients rose from 2% to 64%.

A third drug class was introduced in June 1996, with the licensing of the first *non-nucleoside reverse transcriptase inhibitor* (NNRTI), *nevirapine*, which would become a new part of my regiment. Most patients seemed to tolerate the pills well with no problem, and the number of AIDS cases began to diminish.

Within four years, between 1994 and 1998, the incidence of AIDS in Europe sank from 30.7 to 2.5/100 patient years i.e., to less than a tenth. *Opportunistic infections*, (OI's) such as CMV and MAC became almost rare. HIV ophthalmologists had to look for new areas of work. The OI trials, planned only a few months before, faltered due to a lack of patients. Hospices, which had been receiving substantial donations, had to shut down or re-orientate themselves. Patients left hospices, nursing services shut down, and AIDS wards became occupied by other patients.

In 1997, some patients began to complain of a fat stomach, but was this not a good sign after the years of wasting and supplementary nutrition. Not only did the PIs contain lactose and gelatin, but also the lower viremia was thought to use up far less energy. It was assumed that, because patients were less depressed they would eat more. At most, it was slightly disturbing that the patients retained thin faces, however, more and more patients began to complain about the high pill burden. In June 1997, the FDA published a warning about the development of diabetes mellitus associated with the use of PIs. At the (CROI) in February 1998, a number of posters showed pictures of buffalo humps, thin legs and faces. A new term was introduced, which would influence antiretroviral therapy, *lipodystrophy*.

The old medical wisdom was also shown to hold true for HAART, that all effective drugs have side effects. The actual cause remained unclear. Then, in early 1999, a new hypothesis emerged from the Netherlands, mitochondrial toxicity. The dream of eradication, and a cure is still widely hoped for from the beginning, but eventually had to be abandoned. In 1997, mathematical models were still based on viral suppression of approximately three years.

After this period, it was predicted that all infected cells would have died. Eradication was a magic word. At every conference since then, the period of three years has been adjusted upwards. Nature is not so easy to predict, and more recent studies have come to the sobering conclusion that HIV remains detectable in latent infected cells, even after long-term suppression. Nobody knows how long these latent infected cells survive, and whether even a small number of them would be sufficient for the infection to flare up again as soon as treatment is interrupted.

Finally, during the Barcelona World AIDS Conference, experts in the field admitted to bleak prospects for eradication. The most recent estimate for eradication of these cells stands at 73.3 years. Such number games say one thing, HIV will not be curable in the short term. The latent reservoirs will not simply let themselves be wiped out. On the other hand, if the subject of cure is not spoken about, it will never be reached.

Although it still seemed utopian ten years ago, it is now realistic to expect to control HIV for the longer term. This results in huge challenges for patients and clinicians. The industry needs to develop improved pill combinations. Fortunately, once-daily regimens are already available, and a complete HAART regimen in a single pill is imminent. CCR5 antagonists and integrase inhibitors are being developed. They may even partially replace the current antiretroviral therapy. In June 2006, *zalcitabine* (HIVID) was withdrawn from the market, and a novelty for HIV medicine. Other long-serving substances would follow. In ten more years, antiretroviral treatment would be completely different. With increasing knowledge of the risks of antiretroviral therapy many treatment recommendations have been revised. Instead of hit hard and early, today we hear, hit HIV hard, but only when necessary.

The question of when to begin HAART is still a subject of major debate. HIV clinicians are well advised to keep an open mind for new approaches. Those who do not make a constant effort to broaden their knowledge, will be treating their patients inadequately within a short period of time. Those who adhere strictly to evidence-based HIV medicine, quickly become out-dated. HIV medicine is ever changing, and treatment guidelines remain just guidelines, and they are often out of date by the time of publication. There are no laws set in stone. HIV remains a dangerous and cunning opponent. Patients and clinicians must tackle it together. The following describes how this can be done.

Therapeutic Goals

In the daily chaos of CD4 cells, viral load, routine laboratory, genotypic and phenotypic resistance testing, tropism and *Human Leukocyte Antigen* (HLA) typing, as well as drug plasma levels, the ultimate goal of antiretroviral therapy should always be borne in mind; to prolong a patient's life, while maintaining the best possible quality of health and life. This means, that it is equally important to not only prevent opportunistic infection, and malignancies, but also to minimize the side effects of therapy. Ideally, antiretroviral treatment should have as little influence as possible on daily life. Even if a high CD4 cell count and a low viral load are useful therapeutic goals, the patient's condition is at least as significant as the laboratory results.

Management of Side Effects

Patients on HAART suffer an array of side effects. As a result, treatment of HIV infection has become a complicated balancing act between the benefits of durable HIV suppression and the risks of drug toxicity. About 25% of patients stop therapy within the first year on HAART because of side effects. About the same number of patients do not take the recommended dosages of their medication due to concerns regarding the side effects. Patients who report significant side effects, are more often non-adherent to therapy. The patient should be counselled in detail about potential side effects, in order to be able to recognize them and to consult his physician in time. This can save lives, for example in the case of the abacavir hypersensitivity reaction, or prevent irreversible damage, such as polyneuropathy.

Being prepared for the occurrence of possible problems and providing potential solutions improves both the acceptance of treatment and the adherence. However, patients should not be frightened by all this information and the extensive package inserts are often ominous enough. It may be difficult to distinguish between symptoms related to HIV infection and those caused by antiretroviral therapy. An accurate history, including any co-medication (not forgetting over-the-counter and natural products) is paramount. It is important to consider the intensity, variation and reproducibility of complaints, as other possible causes should be excluded before symptoms are judged as being side effects of treatment. It must be stressed that the majority of patients are able to tolerate HAART well, even over years.

Nevertheless, the monitoring of treatment by an HIV clinician, is recommended in at least three-monthly intervals, even in asymptomatic patients, and more often at the beginning of a new HAART, when it should be weekly or for nightly. Standard evaluations include a thorough history, and physical examination and measurement of vital signs and body weight. Routine investigations include a full blood count, liver, pancreas and renal function tests, electrolytes (plus phosphate in patients on tenofovir), which was also added to my drug regiment, as well as fasting cholesterol, triglycerides and glucose levels.

Gastrointestinal Side Effects

Gastrointestinal problems are the most common side effects of 80% of all antiretroviral drugs, nucleoside analogs, (NNRTIs) and particularly protease inhibitors, and occur especially during the early stages of therapy. Typical signs and symptoms include abdominal discomfort, loss of appetite, diarrhea, nausea and vomiting. Heartburn, abdominal pain, meteorism and constipation may also occur. Nausea is a common symptom with zidovudine-containing regimens; diarrhea occurs frequently with zidovudine, *didanosine* and all PIs, particularly with *lopinavir, fosameprenavir, nelfinavir* and a baby dose of *ritonavir*. At this stage of my treatment, nelfinavir was added, now taking me to 14 pills per day, which was quite difficult to adhere to, mainly because I had to carry my meds with me, so I would not miss a dose. Treatment with zidovudine rarely leads to a severe form of gastric pain, nausea and vomiting in the early phase of therapy, in which case it should be discontinued. In addition to the often-considerable impact on everyday life, gastrointestinal side effects can lead to dehydration, malnutrition with ensuing weight loss, and low plasma drug levels with the risk of development of resistant viral strains.

In most cases, symptoms occur at the beginning of therapy. Patients should be informed that these side effects usually resolve after four to six weeks of treatment. If gastrointestinal side effects occur for the first time after longer periods on HAART, other causes such as gastritis and infectious diarrhea are likely.

Diarrhea

Diarrhea remains common in people living with HIV, with as many as 60% experiencing three or more loose or watery bowel movements per day as a result of any number of possible causes, including: gastrointestinal side effects of ART; direct effects of HIV infection on the gastrointestinal tract; other medications and anxiety. Chronic diarrhea (defined as continuing for more than four weeks) can have a serious impact on the quality of life of people with HIV, contributing to doubts and fears about therapy, adding to feelings of depression and anxiety, and compromising a person's ability to maintain uninterrupted drug adherence.

As with all people, HIV-positive or not, diarrhea can cause dehydration and the depletion of important nutrients and electrolytes, including potassium and sodium. However, in people with HIV, chronic diarrhea can often impede the absorption of certain antiretroviral drugs, contributing to suboptimal viral control and, in some cases, the premature development of drug resistance. Excessive loss of fluid can be life-threatening for persons with severely compromised immune systems, particularly those with wasting (i.e., weight loss of 10% or greater).

In patients with massive diarrhea, the priority is to treat dehydration and loss of electrolytes. Other causes such as gastrointestinal infections or lactose intolerance should be excluded. Difficult to digest food stuffs (particularly those rich in fats or glucose) should be avoided and those that are easy to digest (e.g. potatoes, rice, noodles), eaten instead. It makes sense to remember homespun remedies.

Hepatotoxicity

Hepatotoxicity arises due to chemical drug intake leading to severe liver damage. When some drugs taken in combination or even at therapeutic levels, this can cause severe liver injury. There are several risk factors which are said to play a pivotal role in the onset of hepatotoxicity in patients who are under therapy. The prophylaxis for HIV infections are influenced by several factors such as race, age, sex and hepatic drug reactions which are more common in females, and alcoholic persons. Liver disease patients with cirrhosis are at increased risk of developing drug toxicity due to drug formulations or genetic factors in patients under ARV therapy. Liver toxicity is one of the common manifestations in patients undergoing ART therapy and the role of HAART and in *Hepatitis C Virus*

(HCV) which some patients develop later in their years of being positive.

Antiretroviral therapy can initially increase hepatic inflammation, necrosis and accelerate chronic HCV progression. Therefore, many studies propose that HIV/HCV co-infection may augment the risk of developing hepatotoxicity after ART and HCV act as independent risk factors for the progression of hepatic disease in co-infected individuals during HAART.

Hence, it has been advised that patients should be monitored for pre-existing liver diseases and most notably hepatitis B and C before initiating ART. Ironically, in a recent study, it has been reported that use of HAART therapy has shown the beneficial effect on the onset of liver fibrosis in HIV/HCV co-infected patients with advanced liver fibrosis. Despite the improved understanding of HAART mediated hepatotoxicity in HIV/HCV co-infected patients, in addition to those who are tri-infected, like me: HIV/Hep-B and HCV, the interaction still remains controversial. To overcome the above scenario, patients can be routinely checked for basic liver function tests such as transaminases, bilirubin, urea and creatine levels after commencing HAART for the first 3 months.

Elevated liver function tests are common with HAART, and severe hepatotoxicity occurs in up to 6% of patients, but liver failure is rare. Occurrence of hepatotoxicity depends on the drug classes or agents used as well as on pre-existing liver dysfunction. Nevirapine, ritonavir and *tipranavir* have been associated with severe hepatotoxicity. Several fatalities due to liver failure have been linked to nevirapine. Case reports also exist about liver failure due to indinavir, *atazanavir, efavirenz,* nelfinavir and different nucleoside analogs.

Renal Problems

At the time of HIV diagnosis, all patients should be screened for renal dysfunction with a *urinalysis* (UA) and a calculated estimate of renal function. Elevated risk of developing kidney disease: African American race, hypertension, diabetes, family history, CD4 count <200 cells/µL, unsuppressed viral load, HCV infection. Persons meeting any of these criteria should be screened annually. *Chronic kidney disease* (CKD) increases the risk of developing cardiovascular disease.

It is also advantageous for patients with CKD to be referred to a nephrologist for evaluation and possible renal biopsy. HIV-infected persons with CKD are less likely to receive ART, even when ART is indicated.

HIV-associated nephropathy (HIVAN) is an indication to start ART. *Acute renal failure* (ARF) usually is attributable to prerenal causes or medication toxicity leading to *acute tubular necrosis* (ATN). Dosage of most NRTIs should be adjusted for impaired renal function.

Tenofovir has been approved since 2001 and is, like the two nephrotoxic drugs, *adefovir*, and *cidofovir*, both nucleotide analogs. Animal studies showed a dose-related nephrotoxicity. Severe renal toxicity occurs rarely, but a significant proportion of patients develop kidney dysfunction. In one study graded elevation of serum creatinine occurred in 2.2% of the patients. Acute renal failure and *proximal tubulopathy* with *Fanconis syndrome* and nephrogenic diabetes insipidus and rarely *hypophosphatemic osteomalacia* have been reported.

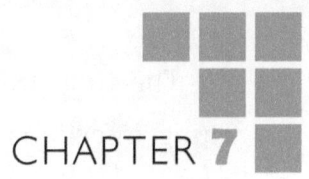

CHAPTER 7

THE EARLY DAYS

Since the beginning of this global pandemic, beginning in the early 1980s, approximately 78 million people have been infected with HIV, and 35 million have died. It is documented that in 2015, 36.7 million people across the globe are living with HIV (40% unknowingly), 2.1 million became newly infected (150,000 of them children), and 1.1 million people died of HIV associated disease. HIV stands for human immunodeficiency virus. HIV is a retrovirus that infects the vital organs and cells of the human immune system. If left untreated, it can lead to acquired immunodeficiency syndrome AIDS, in the later stages of the disease. Uncommon to certain other viruses, the human body cannot rid HIV completely, so when exposed to HIV, even with antiretroviral treatment, you will have it for your lifetime.

The first article, written by Michael Gottlieb, a young infectious disease doctor, and his colleagues, alerted the public health community that between the dates of October 1980, and May 1981, five young, healthy homosexual men had been treated in a Los Angeles hospital for biopsy-confirmed *pneumocystis carinii pneumonia* (PCP). From this information, the CDC suggested, there was a possible link between PCP and homosexual sex and "lifestyle. Gottlieb's communication with the CDC was closely then followed by another from both New York City and San Francisco. A rare cancer in the United States, *kaposi sarcoma* (KS) had historically occurred primarily in elderly males and immunosuppressed transplant recipients. Its manifestation in a large number of young men was considered highly unusual, as was the appearance of PCP in individuals without an apparent cause for immunodeficiency disease. The CDC reported, that 30 months prior to July 1981, Kaposi's sarcoma KS had been diagnosed in 26 gay males, ranging in age from 26 to 51.

It is documented appearance in many young men was mindboggling, in addition to PCP in individuals lacking a clinically based cause for this immunodeficiency. Doctors across the nation, then began to recognize similar patients who had passed through emergency rooms and services since the late 1970s, and it is known, that others remembered many young male patients of which had died of infections that were difficult to diagnose, and that were completely devastating.

The landmark reports in *Mortality and Morbidity Weekly Report* (MMWR) from the CDC only reported a small portion of the story, and the ineluctable evolution of this new unknown outbreak. The reports did not characterize how physicians and nurses responded to the newly diagnosed patients, or how they understood the epidemiologic significance of their past clinical experiences, nor the extent of growing fears about possible new infections from HIV generated unremarkable resistance. The reflection of the healthcare professionals who treated patients, recalled that there was an enormous amount of anxiety in the early years of the infection.

Nonetheless, in the first few years, even the minority of doctors who would then commit themselves to AIDS work had no reason to believe that the dismal clinical picture, that would produce such a grave social burden of epic proportion. Donna Mildvan, an infectious disease doctor in New York who had seen some of the earliest cases of AIDS, recalled years later that she believed everyone was resistant at different stages. In up to 40% of patients, treatment with efavirenz leads to CNS side effects such as dizziness, insomnia, nightmares; even mood fluctuations, depression, depersonalization, paranoid delusions, confusion and suicidal ideation may occur. Efavirenz changes the time spent in several key sleep stages, therefore patients report about persistence of dream recollection and morning sluggishness. These side effects are observed mainly during the first days and weeks of treatment. Discontinuation of therapy becomes necessary in only 3% of patients. There is an association between high plasma levels of efavirenz and the occurrence of CNS symptoms.

Allergic Reactions

Many drugs used for the treatment of HIV disease (including the associated opportunistic infections) can cause drug hypersensitivity reactions, which vary in severity, clinical manifestations and frequency. These reactions are not only seen with the older compounds, but also with the newer more recently introduced drugs. The pathogenesis is unclear in all cases, but there is increasing evidence to support that many of these are mediated through a combination of immunologic and genetic factors through the *major histocom-*

patibility complex (MHC). Genetic predisposition to the occurrence of these allergic reactions has been shown for some of the drugs, notably *abacavir* hypersensitivity which is strongly associated with the class I MHC allele, HLA-B*5701. Testing before the prescription of abacavir has been shown to be of clinical utility, has resulted in a change in the drug label, is now recommended in clinical guidelines and is practiced in most Western countries.

For most other drugs, however, there are no good methods of prevention, and clinical monitoring with appropriate (usually supportive and symptomatic) treatment is required. There is a need to undertake further research in this area to increase our understanding of the mechanisms, which may lead to better preventive strategies through the development of predictive genetic biomarkers or through guiding the design of drugs less likely to cause these types of adverse drug reactions.

Several allergic reactions are quite frequent during HIV therapy. They occur with all NNRTIs, as well as with the nucleoside analog, *abacavir*, and the PIs, *amprenavir, atazanavir, tipranavir* and *darunavir*. Because amprenavir, tipranavir and darunavir are sulfonamide, they should be given with caution to patients with *sul-*

phonamide allergies. When there are limited alternative treatment options, desensitization may permit continued use of amprenavir in patients with a history of amprenavir-induced maculopapular eruptions. Atazanavir associated macular or maculopapular rash is reported in about 6% of patients and is usually mild, so that treatment withdrawal is not necessary.

Skin reactions are the most common manifestation of drug hypersensitivity. These may present with exanthema without systemic symptoms or drug hypersensitivity syndromes typically manifesting as an erythematous, maculopapular confluent rash with constitutional features (fever, rigors, myalgias, and arthralgias) in the presence or absence of internal organ involvement (hepatitis, pneumonitis, myocarditis, pericarditis and nephritis). The symptoms can either precede the rash or occur without it. Eosinophilia and mononucleosis are also more likely to occur than in the blistering reactions. This syndrome has various names including *drug reaction with eosinophilia and systemic symptoms* (DRESS) and *drug-induced hypersensitivity syndrome* (DIHS).

Lipodystrophy Syndrome

The HIV *lipodystrophy syndrome* (LD), which includes metabolic complications and altered fat distribution, is of major importance in HIV therapy. The metabolic abnormalities may harbor a significant risk of developing cardiovascular disease, with as yet unknown consequences. In addition, several studies report a reduced quality of life in patients with body habitus changes leading to reduced treatment adherence. Despite the impact of lipodystrophy syndrome on HIV management, little is known about the pathogenesis, its prevention, diagnosis and treatment. Current data indicate a rather multifactorial pathogenesis where HIV infection, its therapy, and patient-related factors are major contributors.

Therapy and Prevention

So far, most attempts to improve or even reverse the abnormal fat distribution by modification of the antiretroviral treatment have shown only modest clinical success. In particular, peripheral fat loss appears to be resistant to most therapeutic interventions. The metabolic components of the syndrome may be easier to improve, and more detailed information can be obtained from the Guidelines on the Prevention and Management of Metabolic Diseases in HIV by the European AIDS Clinical Society.

Treatment

Treatment should be initiated immediately if there is clinical suspicion. In cases of mild *pneumocystis jirovecii* (PCP) (BGA: PO 2> 70-80 mm Hg), ambulatory treatment can be attempted, and oral medication can even be administered in very mild forms. This may well be possible in cooperation with a competent HIV nursing service. If such monitoring is not possible, and respiratory deteriorate occurs, and in every case with resting dyspnea, immediate hospitalization is advised. If ventilation becomes necessary, patients have a poor prognosis, even today. Non-invasive methods, such as a *Continuous Positive Airway Pressure* (CPAP) may be beneficial if used from an early stage. This helps particularly in prevention of pneumothoraxes.

CHAPTER 8

OPPORTUNISTIC INFECTIONS (OIs)

IN WESTERN industrialized countries, many, OIs have become rare today. This is particularly true for those infections that are associated with severe immunodeficiency, such as CMV and *mycobacterium avium complex* (MAC) disease. The most common CNS opportunistic infections are *cerebral toxoplasmosis, cryptococcal meningitis* and *progressive multifocal leukoencephalopathy* (PMC). Less common CNS opportunistic infections include *meningitis* caused by *mycobacterium tuberculosis* and other fungal CNS infections, such as *candidiasis, coccidioidomycosis, aspergillosis* and *histoplasmosis*. Opportunistic viral infections involving the CNS include cytomegalovirus, herpes simplex virus and varicella-zoster virus. Acute mental status changes can also occur as a result of metabolic disturbances, such as hypoxia, fever, dehydration, electrolyte disturbances, uremia and hepatic encephalopathy.

Central nervous system involvement also occurs as a result of primary CNS lymphoma, which tends to occur late in the course of HIV infection. Central nervous system manifestations of metastatic systemic lymphoma and Kaposi's sarcoma have been reported in patients with AIDS but are uncommon.

Finally, many antibacterial, antifungal, antineoplastic and antiviral medications, in addition to the antiretroviral therapies, have CNS side effects. An awareness of the types of pharmacological treatments used and their potential side effects is important in the evaluation of psychiatric symptoms in patients who are HIV positive.

The incidence of these OIs has now been reduced to less than one tenth of their frequency in the pre-HAART era. However, HAART has not only lowered the incidence, but also changed the course of OIs quite considerably. Infection with HIV may indirectly lead to neuropsychiatric disturbances due to CNS opportunistic infections, neoplasms and metabolic disorders. These infections are unusual in the absence of HIV and tend to occur quite late in the course of illness, when immune function is waning, CD4+ cell counts fall to very low levels and viral load is rising. With the widespread use of HAART, the incidence of opportunistic infections and other complications of HIV infection have fallen dramatically. The identification of the underlying cause of neuropsychiatric disturbance in an individual infected with HIV is very important because some of these conditions are responsive to treatment, and delayed diagnosis and treatment may result in permanent CNS damage.

While survival times after the first AIDS illness were seldom more than three years, many patients now live with AIDS for ten years and longer. One particular study demonstrates this: while 5-year survival after an episode of cerebral toxoplasmosis was 7% in the years 1990-1993, it climbed to 29 % by 1994-1996. This rate has risen to approximately 78% since 1997.

More than half of the patients who develop AIDS today are unaware of their HIV infection status. Due to various reasons, the remainder of patients, with a few exceptions, were not treated with antiretroviral drugs until AIDS was diagnosed. These patients often presented late, usually in a very serious condition. AIDS remains life threatening, and a severe PCP does not become less critical because of the overall improvement in long-term survival. The acute danger remains.

Therefore, every HIV clinician should be familiar with the diagnosis and therapy of OIs, even today.

Although there has been much improvement in recent years, several problems still remain. There is still no adequate treatment available for diseases such as *progressive multifocal leukoencephalopathy* (PML) or *cryptosporidiosis*, and resistance will become an increasing problem with other infections. HAART does not always lead to immediate improvement and may even complicate things because of the atypical course of disease under HAART, as well as with immune reconstitution.

Pneumocystis Pneumonia

PCP is still one of the most frequent OIs. This interstitial pneumonia, from which most patients died in the early years of the HIV epidemic, is caused by pneumocystis. In the last 20 years, knowledge about this organism has significantly progressed, especially through DNA analysis. Although Pneumocystis was previously classified as a protozoan, it was established in 1988 that it is in fact an unusual type of fungus. In the 1990s, it was recognized that every host, whether rat, mouse, monkey or human, had its own specific pneumocystis. It also became clear that the species pneumocystis carinii, first described by the Italian Antonio Carinii in 1910, does not occur in humans at all, but only in rats. The species that affects humans is no longer referred to as P. carinii but is named P. jiroveci after the parasitologist Otto Jirovec.

The term carinii has now been removed from the name for the pneumonia, although the abbreviation, PCP, remains the same. The classic triad of PCP symptoms consists of; dry cough, sub febrile temperatures and gradual onset of dyspnea on exertion. A subacute course is typical. This often allows differentiation from bacterial pneumonia. Often there is significant oral thrush. Weight loss of several kilograms in the weeks before is also common. Symptoms may be even more subtle in cases with suboptimal prophylaxis is rare.

Cerebral Toxoplasmosis

Although the incidence in Europe, and the US has been reduced to a quarter as a result of HAART *cerebral toxoplasmosis* remains the most important neurological OI in HIV infected patients in many areas of the world. Cerebral toxoplasmosis results from the reactivation of a latent infection with toxoplasma gondii, an intracellular parasite that infects birds, mammals and humans. Prevalence rates vary considerably worldwide. Whereas *toxoplasma gondii* is relatively rare in the USA, prevalence rates in regions within central Europe are as high as 90%. Toxoplasma has an affinity for the CNS. Extracerebral organ manifestations (heart, muscle, liver, intestine, lung) are rare and often only detected at autopsy. Cerebral toxoplasmosis is potentially life threatening, and treatment is complicated. In severe cases, there may be residual neurological syndromes with significant disabilities or susceptibility for seizures.

Treatment

Treatment of cerebral toxoplasmosis is not simple. The most frequently used combinations are usually effective (resistance has not yet been convincingly described) but require modification in approximately half of the patient's due to side effects particularly allergic reactions. *Sulfadiazine* and *clindamycin* are equally effective in combination with *pyrimethamine*.

CHAPTER 9

THE ONSET OF RESEARCH

COMPELLING NEW research for this unfamiliar virus began in mid-1981, when the CDC initiated a special task force to investigate the surveillance of KS and other opportunistic infections. The purpose was to confirm that the observed virus was indeed new, and that all the cases were verified, and to determine if KS had previously occurred prior to 1980. The CDC task force queried epidemiologists at all the state and local tumor registries. At the time, the CDC was the sole supplier of *pentamidine*, a drug given by inhalation, which is commonly used to prevent serious lung infections, and PCP in people with acquired immunodeficiency syndrome AIDS. Pentamidine belongs to a class of drugs known as *antiprotozoals*, a medication that destroys protozoa, and inhibits the growth and ability to reproduce. It works by killing the organism that causes the infection. The drug was used previously treat PCP, and the known files revealed the infection had been seen previously in adults without an underlying illness. In August 1981, the CDC requested of all of state health departments to report all suspected cases.

In the first few months of diagnosing the etiology of this unknown virus, the CDC performed a brief survey in San Francisco, New York, and Atlanta of 420 men attending clinics for sexually transmitted diseases (STDs). The Parasitic Diseases Division of the CDC's Center for Infectious Diseases already had become concerned about unusual reports of PCP. The Division housed the Parasitic Disease Drug Service, which administered the distribution of *pentamidine isethionate*. It is in a class of medications called antiprotozoals. This works by halting the growth of protozoa that can cause pneumonia, PCP. Because PCP was rare and pentamidine was not yet licensed in the United States, it was only available through the CDC. A review of requests for pentamidine had documented that PCP in the United States was almost exclusively limited to patients with cancer, or other conditions known to be associated with severe immunosuppression. Physicians' in New York and California had made requests to the CDC to treat PCP in these patients who had no known cause of immunodeficiency.

CHAPTER 10

THEORIES

THEORY ONE) *Amyl nitrite*, (an inhalant used by most of the gay community), was found so very intriguing, that it seemed worth examining, particularly as it was a major component of the "gay life-style" hypothesis that was riveting for the epidemiologic researchers at the time. From 1981 till the middle of the decade, researchers pursued the close association, proposing that amyl nitrite might have predisposed homosexual men to the new human immune deficiency virus.

Theory Two) A second theory surfaced, which was then investigated by the CDC, with the possibility that this new unknown syndrome could be caused by CMV, which is a microbe suspected of both being sexually transmitted and one of the causes of KS. A small clinical study published in 1981, by Michael Gottlieb and his colleagues found a high rate of CMV in homosexual men with KS or PCP, and this group also suffered from a low count of T4 lymphocytes (also known as T4 helper cells). Although it was possible that CMV infection might result from T4-cell deficiency and the reactivation of a dormant infection, the authors of this study preferred to suspect the virus, based on earlier research that found much higher rates of CMV infection in gay compared to heterosexual men.

Theory Three) Furthermore, a third hypothesis came about focusing on multiple factors in which they believed overloaded the immune system, and then led to its dysfunction. An editorial in the New England Journal of Medicine, posited that the joint effects of persistent sexually transmitted viral infection, possibly CMV and the recreational drug amyl nitrite precipitated immunosuppression in genetically predisposed males.

The Journal of the American Medical Association printed an article, by Dr. Joseph Sonnabend, who at that time, treated many of the earliest AIDS cases in Greenwich Village, New York, and proposed that repeated sexual contact with many partners exposed a subgroup of homosexual men to CMV and allogeneic sperm, over time, which led to a damaged and suppressed immune system. He also released another article in the Gay Press, Sonnabend indicted what he called, an unprecedented level of male promiscuity over the last decade in urban enclaves like the Village.

However, he could not explain why the same disease had been documented in Haitians and hemophiliacs. Instead, he then searched for other possible alternative factors, suggesting a list of variables he thought presaged the arguments of future HIV denialists like Peter H. Duesberg, Ph.D., a professor of Molecular and Cell Biology at the University of California, Berkeley, namely, malnutrition, acute viral infections, and recreational drugs.

In the early days of this new unknown virus, the initial focus on gay men and their "lifestyle", posed great difficulties in recognizing that AIDS was also occurring in other groups as well. Among a wide variety of public health officials, there was resistance, and disbelief, to the idea that AIDS could be transmitted heterosexually, in particular, women could infect men. The notion that this unknown virus, whatever it was, possibly be transmitted from mother to child, either in utero or during birth, produced a high level of scientific scepticism from both professional colleagues and the public health community, even with all the clinical and epidemiologic studies. In 1982, James Oleske, a pediatrician based in Newark, New Jersey, submitted a manuscript describing AIDS in the babies he treated, but the readers of the journal quickly rejected his diagnosis. He quoted, "There was such distaste for this disease," he recalled. "How could this sort of filthy disease occur in children?".

Theory Four) It is believed that scientists identified a type of chimpanzee in West Africa as the initial source of HIV infection in humans. Researchers believed that the chimpanzee version of the immunodeficiency virus called *simian immunodeficiency virus* or (SIV) was transmitted to humans, then mutated into HIV when humans hunted the chimpanzees for either research, or meat, and in conduction their research, they came into contact the infected blood. Over the next few decades, the virus slowly spread across Africa and later into almost all other parts of the world. The earliest known case of infection with HIV-1 in a human was detected in a blood sample collected in 1959 from a man in Kinshasa, Democratic Republic of the Congo. Statistics proved that how these persons became infected is not known. Genetic analysis of a blood sample suggested that HIV-1 could have stemmed from a single virus in the late 1940s or early1950s.

Researchers, and physicians believed that the virus has actually existed in the United States since the mid-to late 1970s. Beginning from 1979-1981, there were rare types of pneumonia, cancer, and other illnesses being reported by Doctors in Los Angeles, and New York, among a copious number of male patients who had sex with other men. These were first thought to be conditions that are not normally found in people with healthy immune systems. In 1982 public health officials began to use the term "acquired immunodeficiency syndrome," or AIDS, to describe the occurrences of these new opportunistic infections. KS, a kind of cancer, in addition to PCP, which is a serious infection, caused by the fungus pneumocystis jirovecii. Most people who acquired PCP had already had a medical condition that weakened their immune system, similar to HIV/AIDS, or were taking medications that lower the body's ability to fight germs and sickness.

Theory Five) In 1983, the Cold Spring Harbor Workshop on AIDS held a symposium, and R.C. Gallo, an American biomedical researcher, proposed that AIDS was caused by a lymphotropic retrovirus, related to the Human T-Lymphotropic Virus Type I (HTLVs). This hypothesis was based on epidemiologic evidence suggesting that the cause of AIDS was an infective agent that was transmitted from blood transfusions. It was proposed that it could be a virus transmitted through filtered blood products, such as those used in the treatment of haemophilia patients. The target of the virus may have been the helper/inducer T-lymphocytes subset (phenotype OKT4/Leu 3a+), as the number was decreased in AIDS patients. The only known infective agents with similar characteristics were the viruses HTLV-I And HTLV-II.

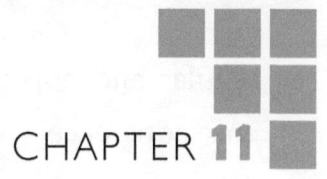

CHAPTER 11

MORTALITY

CURRENTLY, THE life expectancy of people with HIV has dramatically increased with recent advances in ART. The first known cases of HIV-related infections, of the unfamiliar disease, were reported in 1981. The life expectancies of nearly 23,000 individuals on antiretroviral therapy ART were calculated based on mortality rates in the early to mid-2000s. There were 1,622 deaths recorded over 82,022 person-years for an overall mortality rate of 19.8 per 1,000 person-years. Researchers found that life expectancy for HIV-positive individuals at age 20, increased from 36.1 to 51.4 years between the periods of 2000–2002, and 2006–2007, which means life expectancy is now approaching that of the general population.

Antiretroviral medication decreases the morbidity and mortality associated with HIV and AIDS. The success of these medications, however, depends on their regular and appropriate use. Multiple factors influence adherence, including adverse effects of the medication, the number of pills required, dosing schedules and cost.

Patients suffering from *HIV Associated Dementia* (HAD) or other types of cognitive impairment may simply forget to take their medication on a regular basis. Some studies have shown an association between nonadherence and depression, interpersonal problems, drug or alcohol abuse, and legal or employment problems. Axis II conditions, such as borderline personality disorder, also hinder antiretroviral compliance found that, in general, patients who were in psychiatric treatment, in a methadone maintenance program or depressed were more likely to be nonadherent than other patients. Health care workers need to be especially cognizant of the presence of depression or substance abuse because proper evaluation and treatment of these conditions may enhance adherence.

Since the onset of highly active antiretroviral therapy in 1996, treatment has become simpler, more effective, and better tolerated, leading to significant improvement in health outcomes, said Dr. Julio Montaner, director of the BC-CfE. "Treatment advances mean HIV is now a chronic, manageable disease.

Expanding access to treatment to all people living with HIV should be our number one priority."

In addition to extending life expectancy, treatment has been shown to eliminate progression of HIV infection to AIDS and premature death, and significantly decrease the amount of virus in the blood and sexual fluids, thereby preventing transmission of HIV. The expansion of testing and access to treatment in British Columbia as part of the BC-CfE-pioneered treatment as prevention strategy, for example, has led to a decline in HIV-related morbidity and mortality by over 90% in the province since 1995. Over the same time period, the number of new HIV diagnoses has fallen from more than 800 per year in 1995 to 238 in 2012. Along with more painstaking research, the virus was then identified as HIV, two years later, and almost immediately neurologic complications were recognized at a very early stage with this epidemic.

CHAPTER 12

A WIDESPREAD GLOBAL PANDEMIC

RECENT STATISTICS state that 36.7 million people globally are living with HIV as of 2016, and another 1.8 million people have become newly infected with HIV in 2016. It is documented that, one million people have died from AIDS-related illnesses just in 2016, and 16.1 million people have newly become infected with HIV since the beginning of this pandemic. Furthermore, in total, thirty-five million people have died from AIDS-related illnesses since the onset of the global pandemic.

Despite the new advances in the scientific understanding of HIV and its prevention, and treatment as well as years of significant efforts by the global health community and leading government and civil society organizations, most people living with HIV or at risk for HIV do not have access to prevention, treatment, or care, and to this date, there is still no cure. Federal funding for HIV has increased significantly over the course of the epidemic, rising from just a few hundred thousand in Fiscal Year (FY) 1982, to in exceeds of more than $32 billion in FY 2017.

This monumental growth has been driven primarily by increased spending on mandatory domestic care and treatment programs as more people are living with HIV in the United States. Still, federal funding for HIV represents just a small fraction <1% of the overall federal budget of the United States.

In May of this year, President Trump released his first federal budget request, for FY 2018, which includes an estimated $32.0 billion for combined domestic and global HIV efforts. If enacted by Congress, it would mark a decrease in funding for HIV of $834 million, or 2.5%, compared to the current levels $32.8 billion. U.S. efforts and funding increased slowly over time, intensifying relatively recently. Today, there are multiple federal departments, agencies, and programs that address the global epidemic, and the U.S. government is the single largest donor to international HIV efforts in the world, including the largest donor to the global fund.

The HIV epidemic not only affects the health of individuals, but it also impacts households, communities, and the development of economic growth in most nations. Many of the countries hardest hit by HIV also suffer from other infectious diseases, food shortages, and other serious problems. Despite all of these challenges, there have been several major successes and promising results. There are new global efforts that have been implemented to address the global pandemic epidemic in the last decade.

Prevention has helped to reduce HIV prevalence rates in a small but growing number of countries and new HIV infections are believed to be on the decline. In addition, the number of people with HIV receiving treatment in resource-poor countries has dramatically increased in the past decade.

Progress also has been made in preventing mother-to-child transmission of HIV and keeping the mothers alive. In 2015, 77% of pregnant women living with HIV globally had access to antiretroviral medicines to prevent transmission of HIV to their babies, although new HIV infections among children has declined by 50% since 2010. Since three decades have past, and since the onset HIV/AIDS has emerged there have been several lessons that have been learned about this global pandemic.

First, excellent surveillance and documentation of the first AIDS cases were critical in responding to this new epidemic. Second, the rapid identification of HIV as the causal agent of AIDS led to a much better understanding the route of transmission, its natural history, and the wide spectrum of illness. Third, overall innovative science has far exceeded the expectations of most sceptics. These innovations include improvements in HIV diagnostics, such as rapid antibody testing and viral load assays, the identification of AZT, the first ARV drug, the use of ARVs to reduce perinatal transmission, and effectiveness of prevention in many communities through counseling, testing, as well as behavior-based methods, and the development of effective biomedical interventions, such as male circumcision, pre-exposure prophylaxis, and vaginal microbicides, in addition to condom use and needle and syringe exchange.

Fourth, as with most health problems where the etiology is well understood, prevention deserves primacy. Several million persons become newly infected with HIV each year, yet only approximately five to six million persons worldwide have been treated with

HAART. The goal of universal HIV treatment cannot be met unless HIV incidence can be reduced.

Furthermore, as long as the majority (or a substantial minority) of HIV-infected persons are unaware of their infection status, prevention and treatment efforts will be hampered. Finally, our most precious contribution may will be at a time of plague, we will not flee, for we did not hide, nor we did not separate ourselves. The hope for the tens of millions affected by HIV currently and in the future, will depend upon scientists, practitioners, and citizens working together. The future of prevention and care for HIV means standing up to two societal foes, scarcity and discrimination, as much as the biologic challenge of the virus itself. Global resources for prevention and care for HIV remain severely short of the needs. Successful efforts for prevention must also include sustained and visible efforts to combat stigma and prevent discrimination.

CHAPTER 13

WHAT ARE ANTIRETROVIRAL DRUGS AND ANTIRETROVIRAL THERAPY (ART)

A BREAKTHROUGH, IN the hopes of combating HIV first occurred in 1996, when it was found that HAART could durably suppress viral replication to minimal levels. However, HAART was too expensive and complex for low, and middle-income countries, with the exception of Brazil. A massive scale-up did not start until WHO, launched its '3 by 5' initiative and new sizeable funding mechanisms, such as the Global Fund to Fight AIDS, Tuberculosis (TB), and Malaria, and the US *President's Emergency Plan for AIDS Relief* (PEPFAR), came into existence. Antiretroviral drugs are medications used to combat the replication of HIV, and are organized into five classes based on the stage of the HIV life cycle they block. The main treatment for HIV is a class of drugs called antiretrovirals. These drugs do not cure HIV, but they dramatically reduce the amount of the virus in your body.

These medications can keep the virus from eventually destroying your immune system. Currently, there are more than forty-one antiretroviral drugs that have been approved by the *Federal Drug Administration* (FDA), that help treat HIV. In most cases, people with HIV will take two or more of these drugs each day for the rest of their lives. As science has progressed, there are some individuals, like me that are now taking only one or two per day. In order for these drugs to work effectively, patients must adhere to their medication regime, and take the drugs at the right time, as prescribed by their physician for them to work. HIV drugs have greatly improved over the years, and serious side effects are less likely, than they used to be in the early days of HAART. However, HIV drugs still cause side several effects, some mild, and others are more severe, and some can be even life threatening.

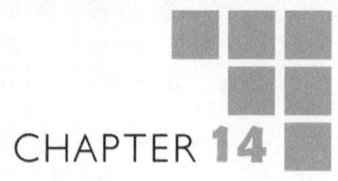

CHAPTER 14

HIV LIFE CYCLE

First, we must examine the life cycle of HIV. Once HIV has entered the body, it targets, and infects a certain type of white blood cell called a CD4, (a type of lymphocyte that helps coordinate the immune response) by stimulating other immune cells, such as macrophages, B lymphocytes, B cells, and CD8 T lymphocytes CD8 cells, to fight infection. HIV then takes over these cells and turns them into factories that produce thousands of copies of the virus. There are six specific steps of the HIV life cycle:

1. **Binding and Fusion:** When HIV has entered a CD4 cell by attaching itself to a specific point, a CD4 receptor, on the cell's surface, it then must bind to a second co-receptor, either the CCR5 co-receptor or the CXCR4 co-receptor. This allow the virus to merge with the CD4 cell, which is fusion. After this

takes place, HIV releases its RNA or (ribonucleic acid), one of the three major biological macromolecules that are essential for all known forms of life and enzymes (proteins that cause chemical reactions) into the CD4 cell.

2. **Reverse Transcription:** HIV's genetic material, RNA, which are the "instructions" that will reprogram the CD4 cell so that it can produce more viruses. In order to be effective, HIV's RNA must be changed into *doxyribonucleic acid* (DNA) the "blueprint" of the cell an HIV enzyme called reverse transcriptase changes the HIV RNA into HIV DNA.

3) **Integration:** Next, the newly formed HIV DNA enters into the nucleus (the command center) of the CD4 cell. Another HIV enzyme called integrase, (a multidomain enzyme, which is required for the integration of viral DNA into the host genome) that combines HIV's DNA with the CD4 cell's DNA.

4) **Transcription:** Once the virus has coupled with the CD4 cell, it commands the CD4 cell to begin making new HIV proteins. These proteins are the building blocks for new HIV viruses, and are produced in long chains, similar to a chromosome chain.

5) **Assembly:** An HIV enzyme called protease (a digestive enzyme needed to digest protein cuts the chains of HIV proteins into smaller pieces. As the smaller protein pieces come together with copies of HIV's RNA, a new virus is then assembled.
6) **Budding:** Lastly, the newly assembled virus pushes "buds" out of the original CD4 cell. The new HIV virus is now able to target and infect other CD4 cells.

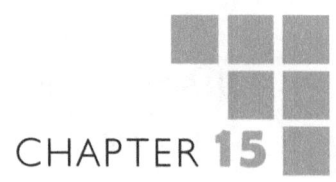

CHAPTER 15

APPROVED ANTIRETROVIRAL DRUGS

TODAY, THERE are 41 different HIV medications: The following list of HIV medications are recommended for the treatment of HIV infection in the United States based on the HHS, HIV/AIDS medical practice guidelines. All of these drugs are approved by the U.S *Food and Drug Administration* (FDA). The HIV medicines are listed according to drug class and identified by generic and brand names.

Entry/Fusion Inhibitors: These drugs inhibit HIV from entering a CD4 cell. There are different types of entry inhibitors; fusion inhibitors, and receptor blockers (CCR5 antagonists), block CCR5 coreceptors on the surface of certain immune cells that HIV needs to enter the cells. One of each type has been approved:

Fusion inhibitor: Fuzeon - (enfuvirtide or T-20), and CCR5 antagonist: Selzentry - (maraviroc)

Integrase Inhibitors: These inhibitors block interfere with HIV's integrase enzyme. There are currently two approved integrase inhibitors: Tivicay - (*dolutegravir*), and Isentress - (*Ralegravir*)

Nucleoside Reverse Transcriptase Inhibitors (NRTIs or "nukes"): These inhibitors block HIV integrase, and enzyme HIV needs to make copies of itself enzyme. There are seven approved NRTIs:

Emtriva - (*emtricitabine* or FTC), Epivir - (*lamivudine* or 3TC), Retrovir - (*zidovudine* or AZT), Tenofovir - (*alafenamide fumarate* (TAF), Viread - (*tenofovir disoproxil fumarate* or TDF), Zerit - (*stavudine* or d4T), and Ziagen - (*abacavir*)

Non-Nucleoside Reverse Transcriptase Inhibitors (NNRTIs or "non-nukes"): NRTIs, are drugs that interfere with HIV's reverse transcriptase enzyme. There are four approved NNRTIs: Edurant - (*rilpivirine*), Intelence - (*etravirine* or ETR), Rescriptor (*delavirdine*), Sustiva - (*efavirenz*), and Viramune - (*nevirapine*)

Protease Inhibitors (PIs): These drugs also help interfere with HIV's protease enzyme, that HIV uses to make copies of itself. There are eight approved PIs:

Aptivus - (*tipranivir*), Crixivan - (*indinavir*), Invirase - (*saquinavir*), Lexiva - (*fosamprenavir*), Norvir - (*ritonavir*), Prezista - (darunavir), Reyataz - (*atazanavir*), and Viracept - (*nelfinavir*)

Post-Attachment Inhibitors: Post-attachment inhibitors block CD4 receptors on the surface of immune cells that HIV uses to enter the cells. There is one approved PAH.

Trogarzo - (*ibalizumab*)

Fixed-Dose Combinations: There also are fixed-dose drugs that combine two or more HIV drugs from one or more classes in just one pill. This can make dosing much easier. There are twenty combination pills approved: (Atripla - (*efaverinz, emtricitabine, and disoproxil*), Combivir - (*lamivudine and zidovudine*), Complera - (*emtricitabine, rilpivirine and tonofovir disoproxil*), Descovy - (*emtricitabine, and tenofovir disoprixal*) - Epzicom - (*abacavir and lamivudine*), Evotaz - (*atanzavir and cobicistat*), Genvoya - (*elitegravir, cobicistat, emtriciabine, alafenamide fumarate)*, Odefsey -(*emtricitabine, rilpivirine and tenofovir*), Prezcobix - (*darunayir and cobicistat*), Stribild - (*elvitegravir, cobocostat, emtricitabine, and tenofovir disoproxil fumarate*), Triumeq - (*abacavir, dolutegravir, and lamivudine*), Trizivir - (*abacavir, lamivudine and zidovudine*), Truvada - (*emtricitabine and disoproxilfumarate*), Kaletra – (*lopinavir and ritonavir)*, Cimduo - (*lamivudine and disoproxil fumarate*), Biktarvy - (*bictegravir, emtricitabine, and tenofovir alafenamide*), Symtuza - (*darunavir, cobicistat, emtricitabine and tenofovir alafenamide*), Jaluca - (*dolutegravir and rilpivirine*), Symfi - (*efaverinz, lamivudine and tenofovir disoprizail fumarate*).

Boosting Agents: The following last two drugs do not affect HIV's lifecycle, but they improve the level of the other drugs in the blood stream, so that the other HIV drugs can be taken at a lower dose. (Norvir - *(ritonavir)*, and Tybost - *(cobicistat)*.

Currently, the previous six classes of HIV drugs target four of the steps of HIV's lifecycle. Attacking HIV by combining drugs from different classes has proved the way to slow or stop HIV reproduction. It is also the best way to prevent the development of drug resistance. Moreover, the approval of new classes of HIV drugs, and new drugs in the classes already available, will hopefully continue to provide more treatment options for those living with HIV in the near future.

CHAPTER 16

HIV AND PSYCHIATRIC DISORDERS

NEUROPSYCHIATRIC DISORDERS, and symptoms still remain prevalent since the earliest reports of HIV. Psychiatric disorders occur frequently in HIV-infected patients, but the reported prevalence rates differ considerably, depending on the stage of infection and study population. Fact is, though, there are multiple factors that can have an impact on comorbid psychiatric illness: psychiatric disorders, e.g. substance abuse, can be an independent risk factor for HIV infection. Furthermore, there are the neuropathological effects of the virus itself, and there is evidence that the infection of microglia leads to neuronal damage due to the excretion of neurotoxins. Additionally, opportunistic infections and some of the antiretroviral drugs may cause psychiatric symptoms.

Patients with HIV infection are at risk of developing psychiatric symptoms and disorders similar to those seen in the general population. Even prior to the diagnoses of the infection, people at risk for HIV may come from certain populations-such as injection-drug users and others with substance abuse or dependence, in whom there is a higher than average risk for psychiatric illness. Symptoms of anxiety and depression may be related to apprehension about disease progression and death and sadness from the loss of health, friends and income. Several studies have found substantial risk for major depression and adjustment disorders with anxious or depressed mood, which may occur during asymptomatic infection. In addition, patients living with an underlying mental illness, especially severe and persistent mental or mood disorders, are at a disproportionately increased risk of developing infection with HIV due to sexual and substance use behavior.

HIV and the Brain

Shortly after the initial HIV infection, the virus enters the CNS and may cause meningitis or encephalitis. Other serious CNS complications tend to occur late in the course of disease, when immune function has significantly declined, though studies have reported conflicting results as to the predictive value of CD4 counts in assessing cognitive and motor performance. Viral load is much more closely associated with the degree of cognitive impairment. Patients with serum viral loads ≥30,000 copies/mL are 8.5 times more likely to develop dementia compared to that of patients with viral loads <3,000 copies/mL. In another study, a cerebrospinal fluid viral load >200 copies/mL was predictive of progression to neuropsychological impairment.

Apart from the affection of the patients' well-being, psychiatric disorders may lead to problems in antiretroviral therapy: adherence to antiretroviral medication be-comes poorer. Therefore, early diagnosis and therapy of psychiatric disorders are of vital importance for HIV-positive individuals.

Medication Adherence, Increased Survival, and Reduced Psychiatric Symptoms

The ability to adhere to a prescribed medication regimen is one of the most important factors in long-term survival with HIV. In addition to poor prognosis for the patient, abandoning treatment leads to a potential threat of multi-drug resistant HIV in the greater community. The higher prevalence rates of age >50 may be directly linked to HAART medication compliance and viral replication. A study showed that adherence to HAART must exceed 95% to limit viral replication effectively. Patients with less than 80 % medication adherence had an 87% virologic failure rate, whereas patients with medication adherence ranging from 80 to 90% reported a virologic failure rate of 47%.

Patients with an adherence rate more than 95% had a 10% virologic failure rate. Other studies have shown that older patients tended to achieve better virologic control when compared with younger patients, possibly due to better medication compliance. Research conducted specifically among older HIV-infected adults reported a significant inverse correlation between antiretroviral adherence and viral load among 100 HIV-infected adults older than 50 years of age. The earliest neuropsychiatric manifestations documented from the first reports included dementia, depression, psychomotor slowing, neurocognitive deficits, in addition to mania, and atypical psychosis. Initially, researchers believed these mental disturbances attributed the psychological reaction to contracting this disease itself. Untreated neuropsychiatric manifestations in HIV+ individuals, independent of age, can promote risk-taking behavior leading to further spread of the disease.

Along with depression, other conditions including dementia, anxiety, psychosis, delirium, substance abuse, and aversive life experiences are all psychiatric factors associated with nonadherence to HIV treatment. Treatment of depression is associated with improved adherence to HAART and improved CD4 counts and disease outcomes. While psychiatric comorbidities are common in HIV-related illness, there are limited data to determine if the neuropsychiatric symptoms are the result of the virus in the CNS, magnified by HAART treatment or comorbid with other chronic, inflammatory illness.

During the earlier course of the epidemic, multiple reports documented that older age was associated with higher rates of seroconversion and worse prognosis once infected with HIV. With the advent of successful antiviral therapy, there has been a reduction in viral load and increase in CD4 counts in large numbers of HIV patients treated with HAART. Studies have shown that antiretroviral treatment can ameliorate depression symptoms and increase medication adherence that coincides with improvement in CD4 cell counts. One study of homeless HIV-positive individuals with depression and substance abuse showed significant improvement in antiretroviral therapy adherence with antidepressant treatment.

The antiretroviral therapies used to treat HIV illness decrease virus production, but may also precipitate or worsen cognition, mood, and daily functioning. There is overlap between neuropsychiatric complications of HIV and HAART itself. Peripheral neuropathy, hepatotoxicity, lactic acidosis, metabolic syndrome, dyslipidemia, and pancreatic and endocrine dysfunction have been associated with HAART. Older patients may be more likely to develop toxicities than younger patients because of normal age-related changes in these organ systems.

More work is needed regarding the complex interactions between medication adherence, antiretroviral drug mechanisms, mood, cognition, and behavior. Future research that focuses on the relationship of long-term compliance with HAART to neuropsychiatric symptoms in older patients living with the HIV virus for several decades is essential for educating newly diagnosed patients about effective treatment of their viral illness and mental health.

Inflammation from HIV and "Accelerated Aging"

There have been widespread discussions of the concept that HIV "accelerates aging," through ongoing and increased inflammation. Once again, using myself as an example, I am 55-year-old, but my body reflects that of 75-year-old. It has been proven, that living with HIV, and long-term antiretroviral therapy causes the body to deteriorate at a much quicker rate, compared to those who are not compromised. Accelerated aging may lead to higher rates of major depression, bipolar disorder, anxiety disorders, psychosis, cognitive dysfunction, and substance abuse in older HIV+ individuals compared to healthy older adults. At the same time, the interrelationship between mental illness and further immunosuppression interferes with daily functioning, medication adherence, and ultimately with treatment of HIV/AIDS in the older HIV+ population. With aging, there are accelerated risks of developing, diabetes, hypertension, coronary artery disease, stroke, Alzheimer's disease, and other immune system-related medical complications, all of which may increase the risks for neuropsychiatric conditions in HIV/AIDS. These comorbidities are typically not observed in the general population until the seventh decade of life.

In contrast, HIV patients present with these multiple medical problems in their 40s and 50s. Over age 50, HIV-positive adults appear to have higher rates of depression and poorer cognitive function, which may be in turn related to changes in immune profiles with age. The common link appears to be inflammation. In addition to the HIV virus, persistent inflammation from other viral infections, such as herpes, hepatitis, and CMV, may activate the immune system in older individuals with HIV and directly alter T cell production.

The immune system has also been associated with HIV and age-related conditions at the cellular level. With normal T cells, one theory suggests that mitochondrial DNA functions less efficiently with age and produces fewer energy stores. This may contribute to the physical exhaustion seen in HIV-related fatigue. HIV-related fatigue is an experience commonly reported in HIV patients over 50 and is often attributed to depression, HIV medications, and medical illness in older HIV-positive persons. Less energy at the cellular level also means lower metabolism for brain cells, which may contribute to a decline in mood and cognition. In patients aging with HIV, this is magnified by the direct viral depletion of the immune systems of cellular energy.

Furthermore, since antiretroviral therapies, specifically the nucleoside reverse transcriptase inhibitors, are thought to decrease mitochondrial DNA, the combination results in higher rates of fatigue, depression, and cognitive changes in older HIV patients. There is strong evidence that fatigue and depression are interrelated. More research is needed to determine how cellular immune mechanisms contribute to fatigue, mood, and cognitive changes in older HIV patients. The role of pro-inflammatory cytokines in the pathophysiology of mood is one of the best-supported hypotheses in the study of affective disorders. Inflammation is also strongly correlated with disease course and prognosis in aging and in HIV. *Cytokines* such as *interferon-y* and *IL-6*, released in the periphery from macrophages and from activated microglia within the central nervous system, may provoke overstimulation of oxidative stress pathways and directly regulate serotonin production and trophic support from brain-derived neurotrophic factor and *Tumor Necrosis Factor* (TNF-α). That deficit was independent of the presence of dementia in those patients. Given the strength of the evidence for involvement of neuro inflammatory processes in HIV infection and neuropsychiatric symptoms, future studies are needed to expand the current data regarding the pathophysiology of HIV infection in older adults. More research is needed to understand the unique mechanism(s) by which neuropsychiatric illnesses manifest themselves in both patients with long-term HIV infection and those newly diagnosed as HIV positive later in life.

Major Depression

Severe depression is by far one of the most common psychiatric disorders observed in all persons infected with HIV. Statistics have proved a wide variation, with 4% to 22% for HIV-*seropositive* men, and 2% to 18% for HIV-seropositive women. Major depression is the most frequently occurring psychiatric disorder in HIV patients. Reports on prevalence rates differ substantially and reach up to 40%. Major depression is a severe illness with serious complications: up to 15-20% of all patients with recurrent depressive episodes commit suicide. Further common complications are physical, social or role model function impairment. Major depression interferes with all aspects of being and may have a severe impact on quality of life.

It is characterized by depressed mood, decreased energy and loss of interest. Patients tend to be unable to experience joy or satisfaction in activities that would usually generate these feelings; they may feel ill, lack energy and experience a sense of doom. Also, feelings of guilt, a lack of self-esteem and self-reproach are frequent. Additionally, neurovegetative symptoms such as loss of appetite and sleep disturbances with so-called early morning wakening or fatigue are common. Furthermore, depressed patients describe somatic symptoms such as pain or vertigo. Quite often, the severity of symptoms can change during the day, with greater severity in the morning and relief in the evening. Poor concentration and cognitive impairment, the so-called pseudodementia in depression may also occur. Depressive illness in the elderly with HIV still remains underdiagnosed and undertreated in medical clinics. This is in part because older patients with HIV often present with somatic complaints, anger, and irritability instead of low mood. Because older patients with depression and HIV are more somatically focused, it may be difficult to delineate HIV symptoms from *major depressive disorder* (MDD). Poor sleep, changes in appetite, lack of motivation, decreased concentration, fatigue, and weight loss are overlapping symptoms in both HIV and MDD. This misinterpretation of symptoms in older HIV-infected older adults may contribute to the delay in the diagnosis and treatment of MDD, allowing the depression to have an insidious course until identified. More comprehensive measures have been implemented in HIV-infected older adults to capture what the conventional *Diagnostic and Statistical Manual of Mental Disorders* (DSM-IV) may have missed in this special patient population. One example is that by using more formal and descriptive methods of diagnosis, one group was able to accurately identify depression, cognitive symptoms, and alcohol abuse with increasing age in HIV populations. Suicide, the most significant risk associated with depression, has been understudied in older HIV-infected patients.

The limited data are surprising, given that older people have the highest rate of completed suicide and persons with HIV/AIDS and depression are more vulnerable to thoughts of suicide, given perceived lack of social support and higher ratings of emotional stress. One survey of a group of 113 individuals, all older than age 45 years of age utilizing HIV/AIDS services reported thoughts, and fantasies of taking their own life in the previous week in 27% of the respondents. Much greater levels of emotional distress, anxiety and poorer health-related quality of life was in correlation with increased suicidal thoughts in this older, HIV-positive group, and long-term survivors.

Many increased suicidal thoughts and behaviors have also been noted and associated with lower CD4 counts and higher viral loads within this group and the cycle of reinforcement between depression, anxiety and HIV illness is further exacerbated by self-defeating behaviors often seen in this patient population.

Treatment

Treatment of depression is based on two basic principles: medication and psychotherapy. In general, treatment of depressed HIV-infected patients does not differ much from that of other patients. Various studies show that antidepressant medication is efficacious in treating depression among depressed, HIV-positive individuals. Medication should therefore always be part of a therapeutic regimen. The pharmacological treatment of depression in older people with HIV/AIDS has not been extensively studied, and there are no specific treatment guidelines.

We do know that antiretroviral therapy may have important interactions with *selective serotonin reuptake inhibitors* (SSRIs), tricyclic antidepressants, and *benzodiazepines* that are commonly used to manage depression in HIV patients. HIV patients should be counseled regarding the benefit of antidepressant treatment but should also be aware of potential interactions with their HAART therapy and the need for close monitoring of medication dosages. It should consist of acute phase therapy, maintenance therapy and prophylaxis of a relapse of depression. The goal of treatment should be the complete remission of depressive symptoms. After alleviation, treatment should be continued for at least six months. At the end of treatment, medication should be reduced slowly over a period of weeks, or months.

CHAPTER 17

PSYCHIATRIC MANIFESTATIONS WITH HIV AND (ART)

RECOGNIZING PSYCHIATRIC manifestations with HIV can be quite complicated with the complex biologic, psychological and social circumstances in conjunction of this disease, and psychiatric symptoms often go unrecognized and untreated. Psychiatric disorders in HIV patients ranges widely, depending on the targeted infected risk group, the criteria for the evaluation, and what stage of the HIV disease.

Depression

As stated previously, depression is one of the most common psychiatric complications of having chronic medical illnesses. Studies have shown a prevalence of depression in HIV patients is two to three times higher than in the general population. Major depression has a profound effect on the use of and adherence to HAART among patients with HIV patients. Having HIV infection and psychiatric illness share many features, and each is a significant risk factor for the other. Major depression in HIV positive patients, is noted to be ~30% and a prevalence of HIV infection among people with severe mental illness is 4.0%–22.9%.

Treatment

Whereas depression is increasingly recognized as a cause of increased morbidity and mortality in many chronic medical illnesses, it remains undiagnosed and untreated in the HIV-infected population. In the context of HIV infection, the diagnosis of depressive disorders can be even more challenging because many vegetative symptoms of depression (e.g., fatigue, pain, anorexia and insomnia) are observed in many patients throughout the course of their HIV illness, even when depression is not present. However, in both the early and late phases of HIV disease, these symptoms correlate more closely with a mood disorder (when present) than with clinical correlates of infection. The prominence of diminished mood in the morning coupled with anhedonia should alert clinicians to the presence of a major depressive disorder and should help distinguish it from demoralization or an adjustment disorder.

Clinical detection of depressive symptoms is even more important given a well-documented decrease in adherence to HAART in the context of depression. Fortunately, recent studies have shown that the treatment of depressive symptoms in patients with HIV infection improves psychosocial functioning and quality of life.

Cognitive Impairment

Cognitive disorders that arise with HIV patients range from mild cognitive deficits to severe dementia, and profound dysfunction may occur in the late stages of HIV infection, although subtle neuropsychological complications have been reported in HIV-positive patients in the absence of immunosuppression. Having HIV can damage the subcortical structures of the brain and provokes a sense of hopelessness and demoralization.

It also magnifies the risk of iatrogenic addictions and potentiates psychiatric disorders. Mild neurocognitive disorder and "minor" cognitive-motor disorder are similar terms used for the early stages of a spectrum of "dementia" syndromes seen in HIV disease. Unlike HAD, a late-stage disorder that we will describe in more detail in the next section, *mild-motor neurocognitive disorder* (MND) may present at the beginning of HIV disease.

However, the symptoms are subtle or may be elusive. MND resembles HIV-dementia because of memory loss, difficulty with executive functioning, decreased fine motor skills, and gait disturbance. These are usually isolated complaints and have a mild degree of impairment. MND is now regarded as part of the spectrum of HAD. With changes in terminology, its description as "minor cognitive-motor disorder" in the literature had fallen out of use.

MND appears to occur frequently in AIDS patients with prevalence rates approaching 60% in the AIDS population. Because the symptoms may be overlooked, the incidence and recurrence rates have been difficult to estimate, especially in the early stages. Current research is looking to whether MND inevitably leads to HIV-dementia. The effect of HAART now confounds this question; data from earlier in the epidemic cannot be reasonably compared with the current data. Early studies suggest that some patients remain stable with mild cognitive and motor symptoms while others advance to dementia. There are not any current markers to predict long-term outcome of the disease.

Treatment

Controversy exists regarding the duration of treatment and outcome of dementia. The long-term effect of HAART on the course of HAD remains undetermined, with some evidence of ongoing HIV-related cognitive damage despite more than three years of potent antiretroviral treatment. The only other controlled trial of antiretroviral drugs compared effective antiviral therapy with and without added high-dose abacavir, but the study did not detect further cognitive improvement. A newer study was able to show some improvements in neurocognitive function over the first year after initiating antiretroviral therapy, but only in neuroasymptomatic HIV-infected subjects.

Antiretroviral agents with and without good CNS penetration, combined with HAART, appear to be effective in treating the virus in the CNS. Drugs that cross the blood–brain barrier and accumulate in the cerebrospinal fluid include abacavir, stavudine, and zidovudine NRTIs and the nonnucleoside nevirapine. Despite these theoretical CNS considerations, there is little evidence suggesting an improved outcome for any particular antiretroviral regimen. However, the higher proportions of patients with HAD compared with other

AIDS-defining illnesses suggest that HAART may not be as effective for treating HAD.

Mania and Bipolar Disorder

Although mania has been well documented in HIV-positive individuals in multiple regions in the world, only a handful of studies focus on older HIV patients. A chart review of an HIV/AIDS clinic showed manic syndromes affected 8% of the clinic population. History of a mood disorder was also associated with mania presenting later in the course of HIV infections and correlated with higher rates of dementia. Bipolar mania that predates HIV infection is distinguished from secondary mania or "AIDS mania" in the literature by age, HIV stage, and/or duration of illness. Secondary mania occurs in more advanced stages of immunosuppression and is associated with dementia and psychomotor retardation. Rates of secondary mania were at one time estimated as high as 4% in some clinical populations, but there are no updated studies to determine if these rates have changes with widespread use of HAART. The general thinking is that mania in the early stages of HIV in individuals with a history of mood disorder and a CD4 count greater than 200 is indicative of bipolar disorder.

In contrast, manic symptoms thought to be related to the HIV virus in the brain in the later stages of AIDS, with CD4 counts less than 200, are descriptive of secondary mania. Bipolar mania and secondary mania should be characterized as different conditions, as they have distinct clinical presentations and management. AIDS mania, unlike bipolar disorder, tends to have a chronic, unremitting course, with the need for long-term pharmacotherapy treatment. To date, there are no studies that look at bipolar disorder compared to AIDS mania in HIV-positive individuals of age >50. One study in Uganda examined age differences in AIDS mania, and this was done in the absence of antiretroviral therapy. In examining 151 individuals admitted to a psychiatric hospital with acute mania, 18.5% were HIV positive, with bipolar mania; 41.1% were HIV positive and satisfied criteria for secondary mania; and 40.4% were HIV negative, with bipolar mania. HIV-positive patients with bipolar disorder were older than the HIV-negative patients.

This suggested that the HIV-positive patients had a longer duration of bipolar illness than the HIV-negative patients with bipolar mania. Like unipolar depression, bipolar disorder is associated with elevated risk of behaviors that increase the chance of contracting

HIV. The risks appear to be more prominent in bipolar mania compared to the general population with a prevalence of 2.3% compared to 0.3%, respectively. The manic behaviors including hypersexuality, impulsivity, high risk taking, and disinhibition lead to poor reality testing and may interfere with decision-making ability and use of safer-sex practices. Patients with HIV, including those age >50, tend to have higher rates of comorbid alcohol or substance abuse, which elevates risks. Irritability, more than an elevated mood, is seen in patients with long-term, advanced infections that tend to have AIDS mania. Bipolar mania and AIDS mania may be associated with delusional beliefs. Most commonly, these involve inventing a cure for HIV or being cured of HIV. HIV-related medication treatment, cocaine, amphetamines, and steroids can induce manic symptoms.

Older HIV patients are more vulnerable to opportunistic infections and HIV neurotoxicity from medical complications, which may put them at higher risk for mania. Bipolar disorder may be under recognized in older HIV patients because of difficulty to distinguish symptoms from MDD or poor recall of illness episodes. In a sub-type of *bipolar affective disorder, type II* (BPAD II), which has milder manic episodes, there appears to be a higher lifetime prevalence in the AIDS mania, independent of HIV risk factors. For example, although the patients with HIV had a chief complaint of depression, 78% met criteria for bipolar affective disorder (BPAD II), 52% had associated cyclothymic disorder, and 35% had hyperthymic temperament. New onset of mood lability and increased goal-directed activity in any older HIV patient may warrant referral to psychiatry for screening and management of acute mania.

Treatment

There is little research on specific treatment recommendations for bipolar mania and AIDS mania in older HIV individuals. The treatment involves management of mania symptoms with antipsychotic medication and suppression of systemic viral load with antiretroviral medications. Older HIV patients may be sensitive to *extrapyramidal symptoms* (EPS) and anticholinergic agents, where medication toxicity and drug interactions are also a problem with increased age. Very low doses of a single typical or atypical neuroleptic medication is preferable for late-stage AIDS mania as they can be dosed once daily, have a lower side effect profile, and are generally well tolerated and maintain compliance.

The most common *atypical neuroleptics*, which are also approved for older HIV-positive patients, are: *quetiapine, risperidone, olanzapine,* and *aripiprazole*. Mood stabilizers, such as lithium, the mainstay of treatment in bipolar disorder, can be problematic in HIV patients with mania, because serum drug levels need to be closely monitored and may be affected by HAART medications. There is also a risk of CNS toxicity if levels are supratherapeutic. Another mood stabilizer, valproic acid, has been associated with liver toxicity and bone marrow suppression in immunocompromised patients.

The long-term use of antiretroviral therapy would be expected to decrease the incidence of AIDS mania in the population and potentially prevent relapse in individual patients. However, more research is needed to determine if AIDS mania rates are increasing as more long-term survivors of HIV age with the virus.

Therefore, an exact 672 HIV and psychiatric disorders history of medication, and especially recent changes in medication are of vital interest. The occurring delusional themes are numerous, including somatic delusions, delusions of grandeur, religious delusions, and, most frequently, paranoia or persecutory delusions. Diseases that affect subcortical structures or the temporal lobes are more frequently associated with delusions than others. In hallucinations, every sensory quality (auditory, visual, olfactory, gustatory or tactile) might be affected.

Patients with a previously undiagnosed general medical condition, such as HIV-infection, can develop an acute psychiatric condition due to HIV encephalopathy, a brain damage from an opportunistic CNS infection such as toxoplasmosis, neoplasms involving the CNS, or metabolic dysfunction. In all acute psychotic disorders, a magnetic resonance image of the brain, and examination of cerebral spinal fluid should therefore be carried out as soon as possible. HIV infection does not show any specific psycho-pathological findings.

Anxiety Disorders

Anxiety is also quite common in HIV patients. Individuals with a pre-existing disorder are at more risk for exacerbation of anxiety symptoms, due to the immeasurable stresses of having HIV, great concern over the possible progression of the disease and the impact it may have on social status, family, work and friends, in addition to existential concerns all may result in more significant anxiety.

Feelings of anxiety are a normal, healthy response to the diagnosis, onset, or progression of HIV infection. But it's important to recognize the difference between this type of anxiety and the sort that signals a clinical disorder. HIV itself does not cause anxiety disorders, but HIV+ people tend to experience more anxiety than the general population. Certain medications used to treat HIV can also cause anxiety symptoms.

Fortunately, anxiety disorders are among the most treatable of psychiatric conditions and respond well to pharmacological and nonpharmacological treatment. Anxiety is one of the co-morbidities that are often overlooked in treating patients for HIV/AIDS. Anxiety is higher among HIV/AIDS than the general population. Anxiety among those that have recently been diagnosed with, HIV has been shown to be more prevalent among patients with stress or excess social stigma related to their diagnosis.

While anxiety disorders are the most common of all psychiatric disorders in the general population, there is far less research in HIV-positive patients compared to mood and psychotic disorders. One review estimates anxiety is rated up to 38% in the general HIV population, but no specific studies have looked at rates of anxiety in older HIV patients or in those with advanced stages of HIV. Anxiety was a strong independent predictor of sexual risk and substance use in one study of 302 substance-using, HIV-negative, and unknown-status gay/bisexual men at risk for HIV infection. Age appeared to be a moderating factor for anxiety and sex-risk outcomes, where older and more anxious participants had more frequent instances of sexual risk. Anxiety that develops from stressors that develop during HIV treatment and pre-existing generalized anxiety disorder, panic disorder, and/or post-traumatic stress disorder has been reported in individuals with HIV.

Those diagnoses with HIV had higher rates of GAD, than simple phobias, with social anxiety common in both groups. Rates of GAD, *panic disorder* (PD), and combined GAD and PD were estimated to be 15.8, 10.5, and 5%, respectively, in an older review of a nationwide analysis of HIV-positive individuals. Women with HIV tend to report higher rates of anxiety. Subsequently, the HIV literature on anxiety disorders tends to be gender specific.

One study used the Hamilton Depression Rating Scale and the Hamilton Anxiety Rating Scale to compare anxiety symptoms in 93 HIV-seropositive women and 62 seronegative women in a clinic setting.

There was no significant between-group difference in the rate of anxiety disorders. However, HIV-seropositive women had significantly higher anxiety symptom scores, over two times higher, compared to seronegative women. HIV-positive women reported higher rates of GAD, bereavement, and suicidal thoughts compared to HIV-positive men after the death of a loved one.

HIV-positive women have more exposure to trauma-related disorders and *posttraumatic stress disorder* (PTSD), with PTSD rates as high as 42%. In one study of 61 HIV-positive homosexual/bisexual men assessed for posttraumatic stress disorder in response to HIV infection, 30% met criteria for PTSD in response to HIV diagnosis. PTSD has an onset greater than 6 months after initial HIV infection diagnosis in over one third of the cases but was also significantly associated with a pre-HIV history of PTSD from non-HIV causes.

The presence of PTSD, GAD, and panic disorder affects the treatment and management of HIV. PTSD and anxiety have been proposed to interfere with adherence to antiretroviral treatment, but other studies suggest the association is due to depression more so than anxiety, particularly in those aging with HIV. Middle-age and older individuals with HIV and suicidal thoughts also reported greater symptoms of anxiety, somatization, hostility, and interpersonal sensitivity. Higher stress ratings in these older HIV/AIDS patients tended to correspond with fewer social support, more feelings of stigma related to diagnosis, and higher rates of social isolation. Anxiety symptoms are common among patients dealing with a new diagnosis of HIV, and clinicians should be aware that individuals are vulnerable to acute stress disorder and changes in mood after receiving the diagnosis.

Treatment

There are three different methods used to successfully treat anxiety and psychotic disorders: pharmacological, nonpharmacological, or a combination of the two. Each patient's experience of an anxiety disorder is unique and must be treated as such. Although many anti-anxiety medications are effective, there are also a number of good nonpharmacological treatments to choose from. When someone suffering from anxiety disorder is already taking a variety of medications, or there is concern about potential complications or interactions between medications, it may be preferable to pursue a nonpharmacological approach.

Medications used to treat anxiety disorders include SSRIs; benzodiazepines, the most commonly used, but potentially causing withdrawal symptoms when stopped; *venlafaxine*; and *buspirone*. Other anti-anxiety agents that can be effective include antihistamines, beta-adrenergic blocking agents, neuroleptics, tricyclic antidepressants. It is important to consider drug-drug interactions and potential side effects if the treating physician chooses to treat anxiety with one of these medications. Nonpharmacological treatments of HIV-related anxiety include muscle relaxation, behavioral therapies, acupuncture, meditation techniques, self-hypnosis and individual imagery psychotherapy, cognitive-behavioral therapy, psychoeducation, aerobic exercise, and supportive group therapy.

As with organic psychosis, the causative general medical condition must be treated first, in primary psychosis, according to its multifactorial etiology, therapy should consist of a combination of pharmacological, psychotherapeutic, psycho-educational, and sociopsychiatric intervention. Symptomatic treatment with neuroleptics is initially the most important part of treatment in the acute phase of primary psychotic disorders. The pharmacological treatment of HIV patients does not differ much from that of other populations, but it should be started at low doses and titrated cautiously, since a dysfunction of the blood brain barrier and consequently a higher rate of medication side effects is to be expected: start low and go slowly.

In acute psychotic disorder, regardless of the etiology, the use of a conventional antipsychotic agent, e.g. haloperidol 5 mg PO or IM, is usually successful. For additional sedation in cases with more severe agitation, comedication with a benzodiazepine is possible. When aggressive behavior is present, *diazepam* 5 to 10 mg PO or IM is a good choice; if fear or anxiety is the leading symptom, *lorazepam* up to 2.5 mg is indicated.

In the further course of treatment, change to an atypical anti-psychotic agent is highly recommended. In less acute symptomatic psychotic disorders, and in primary comorbid psychosis the use of atypical antipsychotic agents is again the treatment of choice, due to various reasons: atypical antipsychotic agents cause significantly less EPS and TD, than typical antipsychotic drugs.

Furthermore, they might provide an advantage in non-responding patients and in the treatment of negative symptoms: sociality, the withdrawal from relationships; avolition, the loss of initiative and drive; affective flattening or inappropriateness; alogia, a poverty of speech production and content; anhedonia, difficulty experiencing pleasure. These are often the most debilitating symptoms in psychotic disorders. Because of the lower risk of developing EPS and TD for which HIV-infected patients are more susceptible than others and treatment with atypical antipsychotic agents might improve adherence to psychopharmacological treatment of anxiety and psychotic disorders too. In case of insufficient effectiveness, a different atypical antipsychotic agent should be selected after approximately four weeks.

Major episodes of mania have also been documented with the progression of HIV infection. In early stages of HIV infection, 1%–2% of patients experienced manic episodes, which is only slightly higher than the rate of the general population. Psychosis has also been highly documented, relative to the mood disorders, and uncommon psychiatric manifestation of having AIDS. Even with the implementation of antiretroviral therapy, it still may precipitate common episodes of psychosis.

AIDS-related complications of the central nervous system CNS can be caused directly by the HIV virus itself, especially in older persons, by certain cancers and opportunistic infections, (illnesses caused by fungi bacteria, and other viruses, or by toxic effects of the drugs used to treat these symptoms. HAD and ADC, occurs primarily in persons with advanced HIV infection. Symptoms may include encephalitis (inflammation of the brain), behavioral changes, and a slow but gradual decline in cognitive function, including trouble with concentration, memory, and attention.

Higher rates of mania episodes have also been noted with the progression of HIV infection. In the early stages of HIV, 1%–2% of patients experience manic episodes, slightly higher than the rate in the general population. However, after the onset of AIDS, 4%–8% of patients appear to experience more induced mania. Around the time of onset of AIDS, this increase of mania is associated with cognitive changes and dementia and is thought to be a secondary manic syndrome due to CNS infection of HIV.

Even with all the benefits of ART, and inhibiting the replication of HIV, there have been several reports of mania in patients treated with zidovudine, and several case reports document manic episodes while taking this drug, even in patients with no prior psychiatric history. In some cases, the patients' mania was severe enough to even require hospitalisation. Over the last few years, fewer problems have been reported, mostly because zidovudine is now being administered in lower doses, at approximately 600 mg/day or 300 mg bid, versus the 2000 mg/day doses used in the pre-HAART era. Moreover, in patients with HIV, psychiatric disorders increase the risk of non-adherence to HARRT, and for also transmitting the disease.

Treatment

For acute mania or mixed states, the mainstays of treatment are mood stabilizers and antipsychotic medicines. Treatment of mania may require consultation and may be beyond the scope of most primary medical clinicians. Mood stabilizers used for this condition include lithium salts and anticonvulsant agents. Lithium should be titrated carefully to a therapeutic serum level, and trough levels should be checked after 4 full days on any given dose. Lithium is the best-studied of all the mood-stabilizing agents, but it carries with it some significant risks due to a narrow therapeutic window. Common side effects of lithium include nausea, diarrhea, increased urine output, weight gain, and dose-related tremor. With prolonged administration of high levels of the drug, lithium is toxic to kidneys, may cause *diabetes insipidus,* and is toxic to the thyroid, causing hypothyroidism. Use of *lithium* in patients with the sick sinus syndrome is contraindicated. Finally, lithium can cause or worsen delirium, and great care should be taken when it is used to treat patients who have pre-existing cognitive deficits.

Psychosis

HIV psychosis is a recognized, but usually relative to mood disorders, and an uncommon psychiatric manifestation of AIDS. ART may precipitate psychosis, but much less common, although, there here have been anecdotal reports of psychosis associated with *ganciclovir* (an antiviral medication used to treat CMV), and *afovirsen* (an NNRTI, used in combination with other antiretrovirals).

Psychosis that occur independently if infection with HIV is to be seen a comorbid condition. Diseases, such as schizophrenia, the typical symptoms are delusions, hallucinations, and disorganized speech. It is thought that genetic and psychosocial factors determine a predisposition or and increased vulnerability for psychotic decompensating. Therefore, and infection with a neuropathological virus, such as HIV could trigger a pre-existing psychosis. Psychosis is a cluster of symptoms, not a specific illness itself, which involves alteration of perception and thinking. Hallucinations, delusions, disorganized and paranoid thoughts, apathy, and blunted emotion responses are some of the characteristic symptoms. Patients with psychotic disorders, the most severe symptoms of mental illness, have higher rates of HIV infection compared to the general population.

Psychosis may contribute to greater morbidity and mortality in patients with HIV by interfering with reality testing, creating barriers to medication compliance, difficulty with communicating symptoms to the clinician, and minimization of HIV symptom severity on the part of clinical staff. To date, aging, HIV, and psychosis have only been circumstantially studied with mainly indirect evidence regarding prevalence, clinical course, and treatment in HIV-seropositive populations with these three confounding factors. Older HIV patients have been studied with regard to sub classification of psychotic disorder; primary associated with ongoing schizophrenia, mood disorders, and substance abuse and dependence and secondary, associated with new-onset symptoms during HIV infection. Schizophrenia, schizoaffective disorder, and bipolar disorder are pre-existing mental disorders that are part of a spectrum of psychosis and seen in HIV seropositivity. This group of patients appears to be more vulnerable to higher rates of HIV infection compared to the general population. Psychotic patients may be paranoid about medication side effects or may be too confused to follow a medication regimen. Subjective evidence has suggested an adverse impact of HIV disease because individuals with schizophrenia may be more vulnerable to the stresses related to HIV infection and have fewer resources to manage these issues.

Interestingly, in an examination of claims histories of Medicaid beneficiaries with both HIV infection and schizophrenia (conducted before the widespread use of protease inhibitors), no difference was found in the likelihood of receiving antiretroviral medications between HIV-infected individuals with or without schizophrenia. A recent study published in 2011, also based on Medicaid claims, showed that the HIV risks among people living with schizophrenia varied across the eight states reviewed in the study but were closely linked to local epidemiologic patterns of HIV among IV drug users.

Aging may have a direct effect on HIV in patients with ongoing psychotic disorders. A recent retrospective cohort study using the national Veterans Health Administration HIV Clinical Case Registry examined the prevalence of severe mental disorders, including schizophrenia and bipolar disorder in older veterans with access to HIV treatment and medical care. Age, race, CD4 count, and antiretroviral compliance were associated with shorter time to an AIDS defining illness and death. Psychosis in schizophrenia and bipolar disorder was associated with lower survival rates in older veterans. Few studies have examined the rates of HIV in older compared to younger adults with pre-existing psychotic disorders. Additional studies are needed in HIV-seropositive individuals with pre-existing psychotic illness to better understand the impact of psychotic symptoms on HIV disease progression. Secondary psychosis, often termed "new-onset psychosis," should be distinguished from an episode of psychosis in individuals with pre-existing psychiatric disorders. New-onset psychosis has been described as a symptom in late-stage HIV/AIDS, with CD4 counts often <200. Common reasons for new-onset psychosis include central nervous system infection, tumors, HIV invasion into the brain, and cognitive impairment.

Estimates of new-onset psychosis, depending on pre-HAART vs. post-HAART treatment error, range from 0.23 to 15.2%. There are no definitive estimates of new-onset psychosis in patients >50 with HIV. Persecutory and grandiose delusions are more prominent that hallucinations. Compared to primary psychosis, suicidal thoughts, first-rank symptoms, and bizarre delusions are much less common. Although the clinical presentation is variable, there appears to be a higher mortality rate in new-onset psychosis when compared to non-psychotic patients. However, with treatment, new-onset psychosis is self-limited and eventually remits in over half of the cases observed.

Psychotic symptoms, along with depression and mania, have been reported as secondary side effects associated with HIV and HAART treatments. Medications, including efavirenz, interferon, *metoclopramide*, *clonidine*, *anabolic steroids*, *corticosteroids* and muscle relaxants have been associated with neuropsychiatric symptoms in HIV patients. Despite stopping the offending agent, these symptoms may persist and require treatment. Patients with new-onset psychosis, like AIDS mania, tend to be older and respond to treatment with neuroleptic medications. Because of age, these patients are often more vulnerable to medication side effects and EPS. The most common extrapyramidal symptoms observed in older patients treated with neuroleptics are akinesia, the inability to initiate movement, and akathisia or difficulty remaining still. One study comparing HIV-seropositive individuals to HIV-seronegative individuals, even after controlling for the dose administered, demonstrated EPS rates of 50–78%.

In HIV-negative individuals with schizophrenia, randomized, controlled trials have demonstrated that atypical neuroleptics were associated with lower rates of EPS and tardive dyskinesia compared with traditional agents like *haloperidol* and *thorazine*. The safety and efficacy of antipsychotics in the treatment of new-onset psychosis have been addressed in a case series, and small pilot studies, but older individuals with HIV have not been well studied. Much of our information comes from the use of antipsychotic agents in older adult populations, but it is unclear if these are generalizable to HIV patients >age 50.

A disorder and brief psychotic disorder can be classified into this group. Characteristic symptoms of psychotic disorder are, prominent hallucinations or delusions. They are caused by an organic disorder of the CNS as a consequence of a general medical condition. In HIV patients, this could be an opportunistic infection, cerebral lymphoma or HIV encephalopathy. In addition to that, psychotic symptoms can be caused by medications or drug-drug interactions e.g. in HAART.

Treatment

Treatment of psychosis can be achieved with antiretroviral agents, and this should, therefore, be considered when cases of first-onset psychosis or confusion following commencement of antiretroviral therapy present. Also, this case shows that symptomatic treatment with antipsychotics can be highly effective. Furthermore, if symptoms resolve after discontinuation of combination therapy, consideration of modified regimens should be considered when re-challenge with the original treatment combination is deemed unsuitable or has been shown to be causative. Although the exact culprit is not known in the current case, any, or indeed all, of the four different medications could have been contributory.

Delirium

Delirium can also be a consequence that occurs during the course of AIDS. Behavioural manifestations may include agitation, psychosis, aggressive behaviour, mutism, and marked withdrawal. The delirium in AIDS is usually indistinguishable, consequently resulting from another serious acute illness. The clinical diagnosis of delirium hinges on the presence of two cardinal features: disruption of attention and disruption of the sleep-wake cycle, which leads to fluctuation in symptoms throughout the course of a day.

A delirium can be easily missed if ancillary features such as psychosis overshadow the core problem of inattention. A routine *electroencephalogram* (EEG) showing abnormal slowing is useful if positive, but a normal EEG is not sensitive enough to reliably rule out a delirium. The sudden onset of psychosis in a patient with fluctuating mental status is a delirium until proven otherwise. The common clinical features of HIV-associated psychosis include sudden onset without prodrome, delusions 87% of patients, hallucinations 61%, and mood symptoms 81%.

In HIV-associated psychosis, neurologic findings are typically limited, and CT findings are nonspecific; however, EEGs are always abnormal in 50% of cases. Cognitive impairment has consistently been described as a feature of HIV-associated psychosis, although it cannot be distinguished from a first episode of schizophrenia. Since substance abuse is a common coexisting disorder in HIV-infected patients and can further impair cognition, it is important to rule out the use of alcohol or other drugs as a contributing cause.

When psychosis occurs in patients with HIV-associated dementia, it is characterized by prominent agitation, irritability, and delusions and is often part of a manic syndrome that has been called "AIDS mania." *Olanzapine* is an antipsychotic agent often chosen for treatment because of its proven efficacy and relatively low risk of causing extrapyramidal symptoms and tardive dyskinesia, which are highly prevalent among patients with HIV.

Treatment

Psychiatric management is an essential feature of treatment for delirium and should be implemented for all patients with delirium. The specific tasks that constitute psychiatric management include the following: coordinating the care of the patient with other clinicians; identifying the underlying cause(s) of the delirium; initiating immediate interventions for urgent general medical conditions; providing treatments that address the underlying etiology of the delirium; assessing and ensuring the safety of the patient and others; assessing the patient's psychiatric status and monitoring it on an ongoing basis; assessing individual and family psychological and social characteristics; establishing and maintaining a supportive therapeutic stance with the patient, the family, and other clinicians; educating the patient, family, and other clinicians regarding the illness; and providing post delirium management to support the patient and family and providing education regarding risk factors for future episodes.

Substance Abuse

From personal experience, substance abuse, and alcohol for (self-medicating), is very common with HIV patients. Obviously, there are several ramifications of continued use, not limited to lack of medical treatment, unsafe sex, and high-risk behavior. Furthermore, there could be fatal consequences that stem from the drug abuse itself.

Sadly, there are people who are more vulnerable that others to the disease, and infection is higher than normal because they will not make reasonable adjustments regarding safe-sex. Since the initiation of HAART, and the superior response by patients with psychiatric disorders still requires further study to determine the reasons for this outcome. It is demonstrated that, among AIDS patients, young and old, and psychiatric disorders, appropriate psychiatric intervention may increase access to HAART, increase their adherence to HAART, and decrease their mortality.

These findings agreed with those of a retrospective study of >1700 HIV-infected patients, 57% of whom were depressed. In their study, they found that patients who were adhering properly to their antidepressant therapy, had a much higher rate of properly adhering to their HAART, compared to patients who did not adhere properly, or were not prescribed antidepressant therapy. Drug abuse is closely associated with HIV infection in the United States: 40-45% of injection drug users are HIV infected, and 25-30% of non-injection drug abusers are HIV infected.

About 40% of people who are HIV infected are associated with IDU, either directly or by having an IDU sex partner. In the United States, 60% of injection drug users are men, 45% are white, 43% have completed high school, and 53% are employed. Comorbidities are common: 30% of injection drug users in the United States are *purified protein derivative* (PPD) positive, 80-90% are infected with hepatitis C, 40% are infected with hepatitis B, and 60% use alcohol. Drug abusers are at high risk of unsafe sex practices. For example, cocaine abusers are more likely to involve themselves in prostitution and unsafe sex in order to obtain money for drugs. At least one third of drug abusers have an overt psychiatric comorbidity.

Substance Abuse, HIV Infection, and ART

Substance use disorders, which are problematic patterns of using alcohol or another substance, such as crack cocaine, methamphetamine ("meth"), amyl nitrite ("poppers"), one of the first euphoric inhalants used in the 70's. Prescription opioids, and heroin, are closely associated with HIV and other sexually transmitted diseases.

Injection drug use can be a direct route of HIV transmission if people share needles, syringes, or other injection materials that are contaminated with HIV. However, drinking alcohol and ingesting, smoking, or inhaling drugs are also associated with increased risk for HIV. These substances alter judgment, which can lead to risky sexual behaviors (e.g., having sex without a condom, having multiple partners) that can make people more likely to get and transmit HIV. In people living with HIV, substance use can hasten disease progression, affect adherence to antiretroviral therapy (HIV medicine), and worsen the overall consequences of HIV.

Excessive alcohol consumption, notably binge drinking, can be an important risk factor for HIV because it is linked to risky sexual behaviors and, among people living with HIV, can hurt treatment outcomes. Opioids, a class of drugs that reduce pain, include both prescription drugs and heroin. They are also associated with HIV risk behaviors such as needle sharing when infected and risky sex and have been linked to a recent HIV outbreak.

Methamphetamine. "Meth" is linked to risky sexual behavior that places people at greater HIV risk. It can be injected, which also increases HIV risk if people share needles and other injection equipment.

Crack cocaine is a stimulant that can create a cycle in which people quickly exhaust their resources and turn to other ways to get the drug, including trading sex for drugs or money, which increases HIV risk. Use of amyl nitrite ("poppers") has long been linked to risky sexual behaviors, illegal drug use, and sexually transmitted diseases among gay and bisexual men.

A number of behavioral, structural, and environmental factors make it tremendously difficult to control the spread of HIV among people who use or misuse substances. People who are alcohol dependent or use drugs often have other complex health and social needs. Research shows that people who use substances are more likely to be homeless, face unemployment, live in poverty, and experience multiple forms of violence, creating challenges for HIV prevention efforts.

Stigma and discrimination associated with substance use. Often, illicit drug use is viewed as a criminal activity rather than a medical issue that requires counseling and rehabilitation. Fear of arrest, stigma, feelings of guilt, and low self-esteem may prevent people who use illicit drugs from seeking treatment services and lack of access to the health care system, which places them at greater risk for HIV.

Since HIV testing often involves questioning about substance use histories, those who use substances may feel uncomfortable getting tested. As a result, it may be harder to reach people who use substances with HIV prevention services. Poor adherence to HIV treatment. People living with HIV who use substances are less likely to take antiretroviral therapy ART as prescribed due to side effects from drug interaction. Not taking ART as prescribed can worsen the effects of HIV and increase the likelihood of spreading HIV to sex and drug-sharing partners.

Cocaine use decreases CD4 cell production by as much as 3- to 4-fold and increases the rate of HIV viral replication by up to 20-fold. In a prospective cohort study, active drug use was strongly associated with underutilization of ART, nonadherence, and inferior virologic and immunologic responses to ART, compared with former drug use and nonuser of drugs. Methamphetamine and cocaine binges are associated with interruptions in ART adherence. A recent national survey showed that 23% of health providers for HIV-infected patients have a negative attitude toward treating HIV-infected IDU patients.

These providers are less likely to prescribe ARVs to their IDU patients even when the patients meet criteria for starting ART.

Treatment

Optimizing prevention and the treatment of HIV in patients with psychiatric disorders, and substance abuse can be achieved by administering appropriate psychiatric treatment that can decrease their risk behaviors, improve their treatment adherence, improve the quality of life, and help decrease mortality. Therefore, patients with HIV/AIDS and neuropsychiatric comorbidities should not be automatically excluded from receiving HAART, especially when they have demonstrated their ability to adhere to their imposed psychiatric therapy, in addition to taking their prescribed medication for the neurological manifestations. The ability to recognize all the above comorbidities is the primary goal of neuropsychiatric therapy. Given that psychiatric illness is present in almost half of HIV-positive patients, at all ages, this is a particularly critical requirement, and of these patients, more than 50% do not receive medication for these comorbidities.

CHAPTER 18

HIV AND NEUROLOGICAL DISORDERS

HIV is classed as a lentivirus, (a slow virus with a long incubation period (months, even years) a family of viruses characterized in part by their ability to cause chronic neurologic disease. It is not surprising why neurological complications of HIV infection are common and not confined to just opportunistic infections. All parts of the CNS can be involved, including the brain, spinal cord, meninges, nerves, and muscles. Neurological disease is the first manifestation of symptomatic HIV infection in almost 10-20% of persons, and about 60% of patients with advanced HIV disease will eventually develop neurologic dysfunction, at some point during the course of the disease. Several factors are involved with the onset of neurological complications, as ART history, the degree of immunosuppression, and the molecular biology of the viral strain, in addition to the genetic makeup.

CNS Complications

Furthermore, there are also difficulties in memory which manifests as delayed recall, even despite the wide use of HAART. Some researchers believe that increased HIV proliferation to the brain is necessary for the development of ADC. Others propose that macrophage-initiated events, lead to brain dysfunction and clinical dementia, even in the absence of a high viral load in the brain. A prevalence of ADC in HIV patients with higher CD4 counts (200-350 cells/µL) appears to have increased since 1996. Moreover, the availability of ART regimens has been associated with a dramatic decline, and severity of opportunistic infections of the CNS, although viral and, fungal parasitic infections may also affect the spinal cord. Systemic lymphoma can invade nerve roots, and occasionally may cause a mass lesion within the cord. In addition, HIV has been associated with a *spastic paraparesis* similar to a vitamin B12 deficiency.

Nerve Damage

Pain from HIV-associated peripheral neuropathy is particularly common and may be debilitating. Peripheral neuropathy is clinically present in approximately 30% of HIV-infected individuals and typically presents as distal sensory polyneuropathy (DSP). It may be related to HIV itself (especially at CD4 counts of <200 cells/μL), to medication toxicity (e.g., from certain nucleoside analogues such as stavudine or didanosine), or to the effects of chronic illnesses (e.g., diabetes mellitus). Patients with peripheral neuropathy may complain of numbness or burning, a pins-and-needles sensation, shooting or lancinating pain, and a sensation that their shoes are too tight, or their feet are swollen. These symptoms typically begin in the feet and progress upward; the hands also may be affected. Patients may develop difficulty walking because of discomfort, or because they have difficulty feeling their feet on the ground.

Treatment

Treatment should be aimed at eliminating the source of pain, if possible. If symptomatic treatment of pain is needed, begin treatment based on the patient's pain rating scale, using the least invasive route. The goal is to achieve optimal patient comfort and functioning (not necessarily zero pain) with minimal medication adverse effects. The dosage of the analgesic is adjusted to give the patient adequate pain control. The interval between doses is adjusted so that the pain control is uninterrupted. It can take 4-5 half-lives before the maximum effect of an analgesic is realized. Chronic pain is more likely to be controlled when analgesics are dosed on a continuous schedule rather than "as needed." Sustained-release formulations of opioids should be used whenever possible. For breakthrough pain, use "as needed" medications in addition to scheduled-dosage analgesics. When using opiates for both scheduled analgesia and breakthrough pain, a good rule of thumb is to use 10% of the total daily dosage of opiates as the "as needed" opiate dose for breakthrough pain.

Oral administration has an onset of analgesia of about 20-60 minutes, tends to produce more stable blood levels, and is cheaper. Beware of the risk of prolonged analgesic half-lives in patients with renal or hepatic dysfunction. Caution when using combination analgesics that are co-formulated with ingredients such as acetaminophen, aspirin, or ibuprofen. Determine the maximum daily dosage of all agents.

Pain

There is also awareness that pain from different etiologies also complicates HIV disease. Patients with AIDS have pain comparable and close intensity to patients with cancer, with similar mixtures of neuropathic and visceral-somatic etiologies. Aggressive pain treatment is one of the most important and challenging interventions in the care of patients with HIV disease. Pain medication has been a part of my life for over 20 years, and I have changed my medication regime several times, in hopes of finding the correct regiment to alleviate my pain.

I have been medicated for overall chronic pain, severe hand and feet cramping, migraines and chronic back pain, mostly due to my scoliosis, which is becoming worse as the days pass and am finding it hard to function properly. A recent U.S. study stated that only 15% of ambulatory AIDS patients with severe pain received adequate pain management. The principles, and treatment for pain in an HIV patient is not very different from that of a patient with cancer and should be closely followed.

Treatment

Treating chronic pain related to HIV requires a delicate balance between relieving pain and preventing complications. Many HIV medications can interfere with pain medications, and vice versa. Also, HIV-related pain can be more difficult to treat than other types of chronic pain. Your doctor must consider the following factors when recommending a treatment for your HIV-related pain: medications you take, including over-the-counter drugs, vitamins, supplements, and herbal products your HIV infection treatment history your history of medical conditions in addition to HIV infection. Some medications may actually heighten pain sensitivity in people with HIV infection. Your doctor may first have you stop taking certain medications or reduce your dosage to see if it helps resolve your pain. However, you should never stop taking any prescription medication without your doctor's consent. If stopping or reducing certain medications doesn't work, or isn't possible, your doctor may have you try one of the following pain medications.

Neuromuscular Complications

In addition to pain, as mentioned, there is also a wide range of peripheral nervous system disorders that can develop with HIV patients, sensory symptoms, and severe muscle weakness. In addition, certain antiretroviral drugs can cause or exacerbate peripheral neuropathies. There are four different types of neuromuscular neuropathies that can arise in HIV patients, which are: *Distal symmetric polyneuropathy* (DSPN), *Mononeuropathy multiplex*, (a type of peripheral neuropathy), *chronic inflammatory demyelinating polyneuropathy* (CIDP), an Immune-mediated inflammatory disease and *progressive lumbosacral polyradiculopathy* (PLP), typically results from the CMV infection, but is very rare.

The occurrence of the above specific neuropathy's increased with downward sloping CD4 cell count and advancing systemic HIV disease. Other known causes of neuropathy are nutritional deficiencies, and diabetes mellitus, which accounts for a small percentage of the neuropathy in these patients. Toxicity of therapeutic drugs, notably *zalcitabine* (ddC) is responsible for some cases of neuropathy, or for progression, however, antiretroviral toxicity is probably over diagnosed as a primary cause of HIV-associated neuropathy. Proper recognition of the different types of peripheral nerve dysfunction is essential for patient management.

Treatment

Although certain neuromuscular complications of HIV, such as distal symmetric polyneuropathy, have decreased since the advent of HAART, HIV-1–associated neuromuscular complications are still clinically apparent in more than 30% of patients. Neuropathies are much more common in adults than in the pediatric HIV population. These disorders can be clinically silent, and many additional neuromuscular abnormalities are detected by electromyography, nerve conduction studies, biopsy, or autopsy. In one study, inflammatory changes, type II fiber atrophy, or denervation were detected in more than half of asymptomatic HIV-seropositive patients without weakness. In another report of untreated patients with mild muscle wasting, inflammation and fiber necrosis were found in one third of patients, type II atrophy in more than one half, and denervation in more than three fourths.

Spinal Cord Complications

Significant spinal cord disorders are less common in HIV disease than are the peripheral nervous system disorders. The neurologic signs of myelopathy, (injury to the spinal cord), such as increased tone, and hyperreflexia (an involuntary nervous system that overreacts to external or bodily stimuli), that occurs in the arms, and legs, have been reported that more than 50% of the older, long-term survivors suffer from these spinal cord complications.

Treatment

The clinical course of spinal cord complications is typically one of slow progression, and most patients remain ambulatory. A more fulminant course may be seen, however, with wheelchair dependence within a few months. Upper extremities are affected very late, if at all. Baclofen (10-30 mg three times daily) or tizanidine (4 mg three times daily) may attenuate leg spasticity and reduce these cramps.

Painful dysesthesias may be treated with "neuropathic pain" adjuvants, such as *lamotrigine* or *desipramine*. As noted above, the vast majority of patients with this condition have normal vitamin B12 levels; however, there may be a defect in utilization of B12. Amino acid supplements that bypass the B12 pathway, such as methionine or *S-adenosyl methionine* (SAM-E), could theoretically provide the "methyl donors" normally supplied by B12 metabolism, which are critical for nerve fiber maintenance. Controlled clinical trials are needed so that the safety and efficacy of such complementary approaches may be better understood.

Intracranial Complications

CNS disorders can be divided into four general categories: primary infection of the brain by HIV, parasitic, fungal, viral, and bacterial organisms caused by opportunistic infections, CNS neoplasms, and complications of systemic disorders. CNS toxoplasmosis is one of the most common causes of intracerebral mass lesions in HIV patients, although its occurrence has declined dramatically with patients receiving PCP prophylaxis, and even further declined with who receive ART.

Treatment

Corticosteroids can be administered to patients with toxoplasmic encephalitis with cerebral edema and intracranial hypertension. Duration of corticosteroid administration should be as short as possible (preferably no more than 2 weeks). The outcome of empiric regimens that include steroids should be interpreted with caution; improvement may be caused exclusively by reduction of inflammation or by response of CNS lymphoma to corticosteroid treatment. Treatment of AIDS-associated toxoplasmic encephalitis is divided into acute and maintenance therapy. Acute therapy should be administered for no less than 3 weeks, and preferably for 6 weeks if tolerated. More prolonged acute therapy may be required in patients with severe illness who have not achieved a complete response.

Thereafter, maintenance therapy is continued to avoid relapse. The improvement in immune function achieved by antiretroviral agents supports their prompt initiation in patients with toxoplasmic encephalitis. Currently, there is no definitive evidence that immune reconstitution inflammatory syndrome occurs in patients with toxoplasmic encephalitis started on antiretroviral therapy.

Headaches

Headaches, and migraines are quite common, and a difficult clinical problem in patients with HIV disease. Although some patients undoubtedly have "benign" headaches, both headaches, and migraines may also herald a wide range of CNS disorders. Headaches affect one in two HIV-positive people, with more than one in four people living with the virus experiencing chronic migraines, according to a new University of Mississippi research paper published ahead of print in the medical journal "Headache".

Severity of HIV disease, as indicated by one's CD4 cell counts, but not duration of HIV or number of prescribed ARV medications, was strongly associated with headache severity, frequency and disability. HIV severity also distinguished migraine from tension-type headaches. Whether there was an association between specific ARVs and headaches was not reported by the researchers. Problematic headaches are highly prevalent among patients with HIV/AIDS, most of which conform to the criteria of a chronic migraine. A low frequency of identifiable secondary causes, notably AIDS-related diseases of the central nervous system, is attributable to the reduced frequency of opportunistic infections in the current era of combination ARV therapy. Disease severity is a strong predictor of headaches, highlighting the importance of physician attention to headache symptoms and of patient's adherence to their treatment.

Treatment

Collectively, the few existing studies on headache typologies among HIV clinic patients portray a very mixed picture that highlights considerable variability of headache symptomatology. Prior studies on headache and HIV disease occurred almost exclusively before the widespread use of ARV combinations. Undoubtedly, the most notable advance in HIV treatment in the last 15 years is the advent of HAART, which was developed in the mid-1990s but not widely promulgated until the early to mid-2000s.

HAART is an aggressive treatment strategy intended to suppress viral replication and slow disease progression that typically involves combinations of multiple ARVs, most commonly 2 nucleoside/nucleotide reverse transcriptase inhibitors and either a non-nucleoside reverse transcriptase inhibitor or protease inhibitor. HAART has indeed revolutionized the treatment and prognosis of HIV disease, delaying the progression to AIDS and reducing transmission, mortality, and rates of opportunistic infections. However, data are lacking regarding the prevalence and diagnostic characteristics of headache among HIV patients in the current HAART era.

Seizures

Seizures can also accompany ADC or manifestations of any opportunistic or neoplastic intracranial complications of advanced HIV disease previously discussed. The most common causes documented are; cerebral mass lesions, encephalitis, HAD and meningitis. About 20% of patients there is no definite etiology for seizures that can be found, despite neurologic, radiologic, and laboratory evaluation.

There above CNS complications discovered over the years in HIV patients, that also include psychiatric syndromes, also may reflect the consequences of treatment with ARV drugs that penetrate the CNS. Zidovudine and efavirenz, are both considered good choices for patients with CNS complications, because they have good CNS penetration, but are both are associated with potentially significant neuropsychiatric complications.

Peripheral neurologic complications including neuropathic pain, neuropathic weakness, have also been attributed to the toxic and metabolic factors associated with antiretroviral treatment. In the attempts to try and manage these neurologic complications, we must distinguish between symptoms related to the HIV disease itself, or the side effects of HAART. Physicians are trying to determine which antiretroviral agents may be causing these neurologic and psychiatric symptoms.

Treatment

Zidovudine, as mentioned earlier, is a nucleoside analogue that inhibits the replication of HIV by interfering with viral reverse transcriptase, was found to be the first agent to dramatically reduce mortality, and some of the opportunistic infections that surfaced in HIV-infected patients.

Zidovudine has been found effective in high doses, in slowing the progression of AIDS dementia, and has proven to penetrate the blood–brain barrier. Therefore, zidovudine has been a consistent choice in the HAART regimens, by targeting dementia and other CNS complications of HIV, although, with this penetration of the CNS, it could also explain the confusion, agitation, and insomnia in up to 5% of patients who took zidovudine for just one year.

CHAPTER 19

THE US AGING POPULATION WITH HIV

HIV/AIDS still remains a global pandemic, and the target population discussed within this manuscript will be people of all ages, but specifically the aging population, including long-term survivors, (such as myself, 55 years old, and HIV+ for 32 years, that live with neuropsychiatric comorbidities in the United States. Persons 50 years and older with human immunodeficiency virus HIV infection, are not only living with the disease, but also represent a high proportion of newly diagnosed HIV infections.

Neuropsychiatric symptoms, like cognitive impairment, depression, mania, mood disorders, and several neurological CNS problems, including substance abuse, are most common in individuals infected with HIV, however, there is little understanding of the relationship between HIV-related comorbid conditions in newly infected older patients, compared to uninfected older patients, and those who have survived for 20 years or longer with HIV/AIDS. In the US, HIV began as a fatal disease of young homosexual men, but today the epidemic impacts people of all ages, including older people 50 and over.

While 50 may not seem old to some, it is often the age currently used by organizations that keep track of health-related statistics. The CDC definition of "older" HIV patients as more than 50 years old but appears to be an inaccurate record of physical and mental health in seropositive individuals. It is estimated that 25% of all HIV+ individuals in the United States are more than 50 years old. People with HIV are now living much longer, mostly due to the widespread use of highly active antiretroviral therapy HAART, but the population of HIV patients 50 years and older will sadly continue to increase. This infected population growth is attributed to both chronic HIV infection from many years earlier, and new exposure in older adults. At the end of 2015, 50% of the AIDS cases in the USA, and 15% of newly diagnosed were predicted to fall into this older age group. Despite the estimated 15–25% of new HIV diagnosed persons in the age 50 and older age group. There is still very little data available regarding this unique population, and very limited data on the treatment of these comorbidities.

Treatment of HIV, and HIV+ Aging People in the US

Treating older HIV patients in the US can be quite complicated, not to say, that only the newly infected, and those who have had the disease for several years, but with older patients, that have demonstrated an increased risk, and severity of these comorbidities. It is a much shorter period from the onset of the infection to the development of AIDS, and present decreased proliferation of T lymphocytes (a subtype of a white blood cell that plays a central role in cell-mediated immunity). Older HIV patients appear to be more vulnerable to HIV infection, because of the lack of knowledge of personal risk, and the low rate of condom use, in addition to delayed or missed diagnosis. Moreover, aging with HIV/AIDS present many new biomedical complexities only now beginning to reveal themselves. Higher rates of neuropsychiatric comorbidities are among the more severe biomedical issues faced in older adults with HIV/AIDS, including widespread cognitive impairment among people that have been on long-term HAART therapy, which could be caused by chronic HIV-driven inflammation in an aging brain.

Currently, HIV/AIDS has shifted form a death sentence, to a manageable condition, thanks to the advent of antiretrovirals in the mid-1990s, although long-term effects of living with the disease and long-term usage of antiretroviral treatment are still emerging. Older HIV patients' ability to metabolize ARVs are severely diminished, and can result in increased toxicity, and the long exposure to HAART may also increase the risk of heart attack, and heart disease resulting from specific classes of ARVs.

Furthermore, HIV+ older adults are at greater risk for dying or contracting new illnesses, such as the comorbidities early mentioned. Furthermore, pre-existing cardiovascular, metabolic and hepatic complications are often exacerbated by the HIV infection itself, immunodeficiency, certain metabolic syndromes, and other adverse effects of long-term combination antiretroviral therapy. In addition to being more susceptible to comorbidities, older HIV patients are at even a greater risk of developing cancer, compared with the general population. People with HIV experience significantly high incidences of certain cancers, including leukemia, melanoma, Hodgkin's lymphoma, colorectal, renal, liver, vaginal, lung, mouth, and throat cancers. HIV can also have adverse effects on the brain, making older adults with HIV more susceptible to negative mental health outcomes like depression, manic disorder, dementia, and even Alzheimer's disease. One study showed that older adults with detectable levels of HIV in their spinal fluid were twice as likely to have psychological manifestations compared to those with no detectable virus. A study utilizing *magnetic resonance imaging* (MRI) scans found lower blood flow to the brain among older people with HIV, compared to normal levels typically seen in people aged 15 to 20 years younger.

Aging with HIV/AIDS has drastic effects on the immune system; each one lowers the production of T cells needed to defend the body against infection. Furthermore, evidence suggests that HIV may accelerate the aging process, and reduce the individual's T-cell count in a similar way to someone who is 20 to 30 years older. A perfect example is with myself, with enduring almost debilitating neuropathy in my hands and feet, chronic migraines, mania, spinal, vision, hearing problems, and severe muscle atrophy.

HIV Comorbidities in Older Adults

Immune dysregulation and chronic inflammation occur much more in HIV-infected older adults, even with those who are using ART. Inflammatory responses continue, due to low levels of the virus and other bacteria. In an uncompromised individual, body inflammation occurs usually in response to an injury, but with an HIV-infected older adult, a chronic condition is hypothesized to lead to a dramatic increase in disease burden. HIV-infected older adults' diseases and conditions, such as heart attacks, and low bone density (indicative of osteoporosis) are much more frequent than in comparison to someone aging normally.

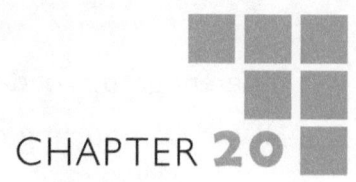

CHAPTER 20

DATA COLLECTION METHODS

MOST OF the research that I obtained within this book was qualitative and quantitative data, which simply put, is research that is gathered through random population sampling, questioners and focus groups, which are performed to minimize risk factors of the formation of a group, that may be different from the general population in which it was drawn. I have also used myself as a real-life example to let my readers understand some of the otiosities of being a long-term survivor with HIV. Statistics are then used to help turn this quantitative data into useful information to assist with decision making that describe patterns, connections and relationships. Descriptive statistics assists in summarizing the data, but at the same time, utilizing inferential statistics, one can then find significant differences between different groups of data, in this case, older people with HIV, by conducting control groups, or long tern control studies. Although, utilizing this method requires large sample sizes for more accurate analysis.

Furthermore, a great percentage of the data within this book was based on cohort studies. Cohort studies are quite useful when it comes to researching a medical disease. The researchers can investigate the causes of the disease, establish links, correlations between risk factors, and certain health outcomes. Moreover, cohort studies look forward to a future period of time. Researchers view the data that presently exists and try and identify the risk factors involved for certain conditions like HIV.

In conduction with this type of study, the researchers form a research question, and form a hypothesis regarding the potential cause of the disease, and observe a large group of people, sometimes for several years, and collect the data that is relevant to the disease, which allow them to detect changes to the risk factors they identified.

In the collection of all empirical data within this book, and to protect the integrity of such detailed information, the main focus was honesty in presenting my own ideas, and ensuring accountability making sure that it meets scientific and ethical standards, but not limited to rigorous analysis, with all the information used to increase knowledge that in no way harms anyone but can potentially benefit society. It is also crucial to report accurate records of the primary data that was retrieved, and truthful in disclosing what was done, how it was accomplished, citing references and the results that were obtained.

Research involving humans may produce many benefits that can positively affect the welfare of society, through the advancement of knowledge for future generations, and, at times, for the participants themselves. In most research, the primary benefits produced are for society and for the continued advancement of knowledge.

Data Analysis

As stated earlier, most of the primary data within this book was descriptive that was used to present qualitative and quantitative descriptions in a manageable form. Using descriptive statistics, one can measure a large number of people. Descriptive statistics help simplify large amounts of data sensibly. Moreover, descriptive statistics are used to describe the sample, and demonstrate how the sample, (aging HIV patients), and how it reflects the population's measures.

Descriptive statistics are very important because if one simply presented the raw data it would be hard to visualize what the data was actually showing, especially with a large amount, therefore it enables us to present the data in a more meaningful way, which ultimately allow better interpretation of the data, however, it is simple to say, one may not have access to the whole population they are interested in investigating, but only a limited number of data, so the properties of these samples, such as the mean or standard deviation, are not parameters, but inferential statistics, which are techniques that allow us to use these samples to make generalizations about the populations from which the samples were drawn.

In addition to using descriptive statistics, some of the data within this book was retrieved using cohort randomized control studies, (studies which are studies carried out over a future period of time). This method is used by many epidemiologists that allow them look at data that already exists, which helps them identify risk factors for particular conditions, and is a way to obtain information about a new, or recently discovered phenomena. In the process of a cohort study, researchers raise a research question, forming a hypothesis about the potential causes of a disease, which in this case is known, then the researchers can observe a group of people, the cohort, over a long period of time collecting a large amount of data that may be relevant to the disease. This also will enable researchers to analyze changes in health conditions in relation to the potential risk factors that have been identified.

Furthermore, using cohort randomized controlled trials enables us to test the safety and potential benefit of a treatment, i.e., HAART, which can prove the harms of this treatment, or also prove it beneficial.

Findings

Over the past three decades, with new research, and the clinical history of HIV infection, physicians have now grouped the disease into three main factors; the widespread use of HAART, which has dramatically lengthened mortality, new therapeutic strategies, which has transformed HIV from a fatal disease into a manageable chronic condition, in addition to the identification of risk factors for side effects, including neuropsychiatric comorbidities. Studies prove a longer life expectancy is already apparent. Since 2015 more than half of the HIV-positive population in the United States are 50 years and older, and most of these older adults were became infected in their youth, or middle age.

Limitations

Presently, the health care infrastructure is ill equipped to handle individually tailored treatment and care needs of HIV+ positive people, and HIV-positive older adults. The long-term effects of antiretroviral use are still being researched and have been associated with a number of neuropsychiatric comorbidities. The stigma with these comorbidities, pose great challenges for those in need of services and health care, which dramatically affects their mental health, and drug regime adherence. Continued research, and several policy changes hopefully will improve the health outcomes for HIV-positive, and older persons with HIV by increasing better access to treatment and support.

HIV and aging with the virus also present many biomedical complexities, and limitations that are only recently beginning to reveal themselves. Much higher rates of certain comorbidities are among the more severe biomedical issues facing these older adults. Widespread cognitive impairment with persons on HAART proves to be caused by chronic HIV driven inflammation of the aging brain. Other limitations, and answers to critical research questions into how HIV medications interact with medications that treat other conditions are still in the nascent stages.

Further Limitations

The long-term effects of HAART and mental health are still very unclear. Research suggests that antiretroviral therapy may increase the risk of Alzheimer's disease, depression, and several other psychiatric issues. The number of HIV-positive people, 50 and older continues to grow in the United States, and it crucial to take appropriate measures to ensure that the needs of this unique population are met. Providers must recognize the high prevalence of comorbidities, and the long-term effects of HAART. The social context in which older adults with HIV/AIDS live, and the damaging stigma affects their physical and emotional well-being, should also be considered in improving care. Furthermore, increased training for geriatric workers is essential to promote the long-term health of this population.

Moreover, new policy changes are much needed, and with these changes, it could improve health outcomes for HIV-positive older adults by increasing better access to treatment and much needed support. A collaborative effort involving multiple agencies and the Government is needed to address these complexities within this unique population of HIV older adults. U.S. clinicians will sadly encounter even more increasing numbers of older HIV patients in the approaching years. Current data from the CDC reflects that the cumulative number of HIV/AIDS cases among American adults over 50 has quintupled during the last decade. In 2000 alone, the patients over 50 accounted for a staggering 15% of all AIDS cases recorded in the United States.

Application of Findings

The use and application regarding findings, results, and outcomes within this book hopefully will contribute to further knowledge, and promote continued research for this disease, with clinicians, federal agencies, and the government in hopes to eventually find a cure. Although, there are several correlations with HIV, HAART, and the HIV aging population, with neuropsychiatric symptoms, the research still remains to be unclear. Since the breakthrough, and creation of antiretroviral medication ART, two decades ago, it has proven to dramatically increase life expectancy for people living with HIV, but with this advance in medicine, it has also created new and unfamiliar challenges.

Whether these complications are due to the direct or indirect effects of HIV, or long-time HAART on the brain, and the effects of these comorbidities, careful diagnosis and treatment are of the utmost importance. Older people living with HIV, and long-term HAART experience a number of neuropsychiatric comorbidities that desperately need to be addressed, if not just for the sake of science, but in hopes, that one day, a cure could be in reach, with prevention counseling, proper screening, and early detection. With much further research, holds the promise of refining existing therapies and the development of new treatment options for all those that suffer from this debilitating disease.

The Center for Disease Control (CDC)

I believe one solid recommendation should be for the CDC to fund social marketing campaigns that address the stigma related to HIV and aging with HIV. These marketing campaigns should target the general public and health care providers to inquire about their sexual orientation, gender identity, and sexual behavior, given the greater prevalence of antigay views and misinformation about the transmission of HIV in older adults, these campaigns should be geared more towards older adults.

To further elaborate; Act Against AIDS is a five-year, $45 million communications campaign designed to refocus national attention on the HIV crisis in America, that was first launched in 2009. The CDC's Act Against AIDS campaign uses TV and radio public service announcements, online, airport, transit ads, physician communications, and partnerships with leading non-profit organizations to reach the general public, and target populations most at risk with HIV prevention and testing messages.

Moreover, to increase, and reach out to the community, the Act Against AIDS Campaign and CDC, work closely with a number of public health, media, and other partners who distribute campaign messages and materials, donate advertising space and promotes broadcasting public service announcements.

Laws

Another recommendation I believe should be to change these prehistoric laws criminalizing HIV, and the nondisclosure of one's HIV status, that only reinforces the stigma related to this disease, discrimination and continued prejudice. There are 34 states in the United States that have laws punishing people for exposing another person to HIV, usually through nondisclosure of their status, even if transmission does not occur. Those persons that are convicted often have to register as sex offenders, which labels them for the rest of their lives. Congresswoman Barbara Lee (D-CA) introduced this bill by in 2011, but the REPEAL HIV Criminalization Act, has since acted to review and repeal such a law.

In March of 2017 Congress members Ileana Ros-Lehtinen (R–Fla.) and Barbara Lee (D-Calif.), once again reintroduced the REPEAL (Repeal Existing Policies that Encourage and Allow Legal) HIV Discrimination Act. Known as H.R. 1739, this bill currently has 28 initial cosponsors. In the reintroduction of this bill, it promises to modernize laws and policies to eliminate discrimination against those living with HIV/AIDS. This bill expresses the sense of congress that federal and state laws, policies, and regulations should not place any additional burden on individuals because their HIV status and is offering a step-by-step plan to work with states to modernize their laws.

It is almost ludicrous that 34 states have criminal statutes based on much out-dated information regarding HIV/AIDS. This bipartisan legislation would allow federal and state officials, and stakeholders to work with one another to repeal these laws that target people living with HIV/AIDS. If it is passed, the act will be a magnanimous step forward towards ending unjust HIV criminalization laws in the United States.

National Institute of Health (NIH)

Another pertinent recommendation, is for The NIH to continue funding large-scale, national, longitudinal studies that investigate how HAART and HIV disease interact with aging bodies, and how they interact with new treatments for comorbidities such as neuropsychiatric conditions, and to what extent the normal aging processes results from the virus itself. Several NIH-wide initiatives are in support for the continued research for medical management of HIV/AIDS in older patients. NIH is currently working diligently towards soliciting grant applications for more clinical and translational studies of HIV infection and associated comorbidities, treatments, biobehavioral and social factors in older adults. Furthermore, the *National Institute of Allergy and Infectious Diseases* (NIAID) has also provided supplemental funding to several of its Centers for AIDS Research on HIV and aging.

Also, a transnational NIH coordinating committee on HIV and aging coordinates various scientific efforts related to HIV and aging. In 2011, the NIH Office of AIDS Research created a group of experts to study HIV and aging, and to assess the state of the science and identify more research priorities. A report in 2012, stated they had created a list of several themes, which will inform the NIA's efforts moving forward towards, multi-morbidity, polypharmacy, and complexities with the management of HIV with treatment effects, aging, and comorbidities that stem from the disease, and a need to emphasize more on human studies to account for these complexities, focus on community support, caregivers and new infrastructure.

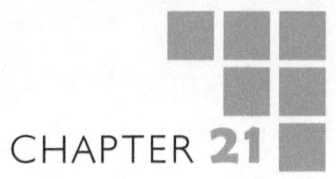

CHAPTER 21

CONCLUSION

THE OVERALL HIV infected population has changed significantly since the beginning of this global pandemic in 1981 and there has been a major increase in the mean age of those infected, and the current overall profile of HIV infection, the opportunistic, and neuropsychiatric comorbidity infections that those infected have to endure, in addition to the effects of long-term HAART, immune suppression, that poses many new questions with physicians, and researchers.

People with HIV infection are subject to the same forms of psychiatric illness and psychological distress as those without HIV. However, individuals with histories of drug abuse and dependence are at greater risk for a variety of psychiatric disorders. People with waning immunity and high viral loads may be at particular risk for the CNS complications of AIDS, such as HAD or

CNS opportunistic infections and other causes of acute mental status changes. The unique biological, psychological and environmental factors involved in treating those with HIV infection require an awareness of these influences in order to arrive at appropriate psychiatric evaluation and effective treatment strategies.

Neuropsychiatric disorders when delivered in collaboration with effective HIV care, has been proven to improve outcomes and quality of life. Successful treatment of HIV, and comorbidities may also allow patients to achieve levels of function they may never have considered to be within their reach subsequent to their diagnosis of HIV. As research continues, and new developments become available to help patients live more normal lives, it is crucial for clinicians to have the skills and resources to assess and manage the disorders that hinder treatment of patients with HIV, and these comorbidities.

This is critical not only in terms of cost containment and outcome measures, but as a matter of doing what is right for the vulnerable, underserved, and disenfranchised patients who currently get and transmit HIV at epidemic rates. As stated earlier, there have been several studies, and discussions about the concept that HIV "accelerates aging," most likely through ongoing and increased inflammation. Accelerated aging may lead to higher rates of major depression, cognitive dysfunction, bipolar disorder, anxiety disorders, psychosis, and substance abuse in older HIV+ individuals compared to healthy older adults.

The affliction of HIV, and HAART implies a multiplicity of neuropsychiatric disorders covering a plethora of somatic and neuropsychiatric loss of health. The spectrum of comorbidities associated with HIV/HAART is prodigious. In order for HIV patients, whether newly diagnosed, or long-term survivors to regain their capability and complete daily normal ability is primarily dependent upon attaining viral suppression. Along with all the issues related to HIV, and HAART, and the neuropsychiatric manifestations displayed in this book, studies have proven that there is a strong correlation between having HIV, and long-term HAART.

Lastly, older HIV patients/long-term survivors, like me, are at a much higher risk of developing these comorbidities, which ultimately can affect their treatment, mental health, early onset of aging, drug adherence, drug abuse, and eventually could become resistant to all their medication treatments. Incorporating patient values and preferences into shared decisions regarding medication regime, adherence interventions, HIV care management, comorbidities, and with continued research, together it will hopefully lead to the best chance of longer mortality, and care for all those afflicted by this global pandemic. And with all this, I'm still here...

LIST OF DEFINITIONS

Acute Tubular Necrosis (ATN):

Acute Renal Failure with mild to severe damage or necrosis of tubule cells, usually secondary to either Nephrotoxicity, ischemia after major surgery, trauma severe Hypovolemia, sepsis, or burns.

AIDS Dementia Complex:

An insidious metabolic encephalopathy affecting up to two-thirds of AIDS patients, which is triggered by HIV and driven by neurotoxins secreted by macrophages and microglia. It may be complicated by infections e.g., Toxoplasma gondii, CMV, or lymphomas.

AIDS HIV-Associated Dementia (HAD):

A subacute or chronic HIV-1 encephalitis, the most common neurologic complication in the later stages of HIV infection; manifested clinically as a progressive dementia, accompanied by motor abnormalities.

Amoebiasis:

Infection with the protozoan Entamoeba histolytica, a pathogen associated with poor sanitary conditions.

Amyl Nitrite:

A volatile, flammable liquid with a pungent ethereal odor. It is administered by inhalation for the treatment of cyanide poisoning, producing methemoglobin which binds cyanide, and as a diagnostic aid in tests of reserve cardiac function and diagnosis of certain Heart Murmurs.

Anabolic Steroids:

Drugs which promote tissue growth, especially of muscle, by stimulating protein synthesis. Anabolic steroids are synthetic male sex hormones and tend to cause virilization These steroids are sometimes misused by athletes and bodybuilders to gain an unfair advantage.

Antiprotozoals:

Drugs used to treat infections with protozoal organisms. Examples are *tinidazole* (Fastigyn) for *amoebiasis, giardiasis*, ulcerative gingivitis and *trichomoniasis*; and *pentamidine* (Pentacarinat) and *atovaquone* (Wellvone) for Pneumocystis carinii pneumonia.

Antiretroviral Therapy:

The use of antiretroviral medications to suppress and limit the progression of HIV.

Aspergillosis:

Aspergillosis refers to several forms of disease caused by a fungus in the genus. Aspergillosis fungal infections can occur in the ear canal, eyes, nose, sinus cavities, and lungs. In some individuals, the infection can even invade bone and the membranes that enclose the brain and spinal cord, (meningitis).

Atovaquone:

An antibiotic used in treatment of mild to moderate *Pneumocystis carinii Pneumonia* and prevention and treatment of falciparum malaria; administered orally.

Benzodiazepines:

Benzodiazepines are a class of drugs primarily used for treating anxiety, but they also are effective in treating several other conditions. The exact mechanism of action of benzodiazepines is not known, but they appear to work by affecting neurotransmitters in the brain, chemicals that nerves release in order to communicate with other nearby nerves.

Bipolar Affective Disorder BPAD II:

BPAD II is characterized by high episodes of euphoria and low episodes of depression, together known as hypomania.

Candidiasis:

Candidiasis is an infection caused by a species of the yeast *Candida*, usually *Candida albicans*. This is a common cause of vaginal infections in women. Also, *Candida* may cause mouth infections in people with reduced immune function, or in patients taking certain antibiotics.

Carinii Pneumonia (PCP):

Pneumonia is an infection of the lung that can be caused by nearly any class of organism known to cause human infections. These include bacteria, amoebae, viruses, fungi, and parasites.

CD8 Cells:

A glycoprotein that is found on the surface of certain T cells, especially cytotoxic T lymphocytes, and that functions to bind the T cell to molecules on the surface of the target cell that is to be killed.

CD4 Cells:

A major classification of T lymphocytes, referring to those that carry CD4 antigens; most are helper cells.

Cerebral Toxoplasmosis:

Toxoplasmosis is an infectious disease caused by the one-celled protozoan parasite.

Chemokine Receptor (CCR5):

A gene on chromosome 3p21.31 that encodes a member of the beta chemokine receptor family, which is similar to G protein-coupled receptors. CCR5 is expressed by T cells and macrophages.

Chronic Inflammatory Demyelinating Polyneuropathy (CIDP):

An uncommon, acquired, demyelinating sensorimotor polyneuropathy, clinically characterized by insidious onset, slow evolution, (either steady progression or stepwise), and chronic course; symmetric weakness is a predominant symptom, often involving proximal leg muscles, accompanied by paresthesias, but not pain.

Coccidioidomycosis:

Coccidioidomycosis is an infection caused by inhaling the microscopic spores of the fungus *Coccidioides immitis*. Spores are the tiny, thick-walled structures that fungi use to reproduce. Coccidioidomycosis exists in three forms. The acute form produces flu-like symptoms.

Comorbidities:

A concomitant but unrelated pathologic or disease process; usually used in epidemiology to indicate the coexistence of two or more disease processes.

Corticosteroids:

Corticosteroids are group of natural and synthetic analogues of the hormones secreted by the hypothalamic-anterior pituitary-adrenocortical (HPA) axis, more commonly referred to as the pituitary gland. These include glucocorticoids, which are anti-inflammatory agents with a large number of other functions; mineralocorticoids, which control salt and water balance primarily through action on the kidneys; and corticotropins, which control secretion of hormones by the pituitary gland.

Cryptococcal Meningitis:

An opportunistic infection of the meninges and spinal cord by Cryptococcus neoformans. Severe headache, confusion, photosensitivity, blurred vision, fever, speech difficulties. If untreated it can cause coma or death.

Cytokins:

A general term for a range of proteins of low molecular weight that exert a stimulating or inhibiting influence on the proliferation, differentiation and function of cells of the immune system.

Cytomegalovirus (CMV):

A genus of herpes viruses closely related to genus roseolovirus containing the single species human herpesvirus 5.

Dendritic Cells:

An antigen-presenting leukocyte found in the skin, mucosa, and lymphoid tissues that initiates a primary immune response by activating lymphocytes and secreting cytokines.

Diabetes Insipidus (DI):

Diabetes insipidus (DI) is a disorder that causes the patient to produce tremendous quantities of urine. The massively increased urine output is usually accompanied by intense thirst.

Encephalitis:

Encephalitis is an inflammation of the brain, usually caused by a direct viral infection or a hyper-sensitivity reaction to a virus or foreign protein. Brain inflammation caused by a bacterial infection is sometimes called cerebritis. When both the brain and spinal cord are involved, the disorder is called encephalomyelitis. An inflammation of the brain's covering, or meninges, is called meningitis.

Eosinophils:

A leukocyte with coarse, round granules present.

Epitopes:

A small molecular region of an antigen that binds to a particular antibody or antigen receptor on a T cell; an antigenic determinant. A single antigen can have multiple epitopes.

Extrapyramidal Symptoms: (EPS)

A group of side effects associated with antipsychotic medications. EPS include parkinsonism, akathisia, dystonia, and tardive dyskinesia.

Fanconi's Syndrome:

Fanconi's syndrome is a set of kidney malfunctions brought about by a variety of unrelated disorders. Kidney malfunction leads to excessive urine production and excessive thirst, resulting in deficits of water, calcium, potassium, magnesium, and other substances in the body. It often leads to bone disease and stunted growth.

Ganciclovir:

A derivative of Acyclovir used in the form of the base or the sodium salt in treatment of cytomegalovirus infections of the retina; administered orally, intravenously, or by intravitreous injection or implantation.

Giardiasis:

Giardiasis is a common intestinal infection spread by eating contaminated food, drinking contaminated water, or through direct contact with the organism that causes the disease, *Giardia lamblia*. Giardiasis is found throughout the world and is a common cause of traveller's diarrhea. In the United States it is a growing problem, especially among children in childcare centers.

Herpes Virus:

Any of the animal viruses that cause painful blisters on the skin.

Highly Active Antiretroviral Therapy: (HAART)

The aggressive use of extremely potent antiretroviral agents in the treatment of human immunodeficiency virus infection.

Histoplasmosis:

Histoplasmosis is an infectious disease caused by inhaling the microscopic spores of the fungus *Histoplasma capsulatum*. The disease exists in three forms.

Acute or primary histoplasmosis causes flulike symptoms. Most people who are infected recover without medical intervention.

Human Leukocyte Antigen (HLA):

HLA typing is used to match organ and tissue transplant recipints with compatible donars.

HTLV-1:

A retrovirus associated with adult leukemia and lymphoma and with certain demyelinating diseases.

HTLV-III:

Human T-cell lymphotropic virus, type III.

Human Immune Deficiency Virus (HIV):

A retrovirus of the genus Lentivirus that causes AIDS by infecting helper T cells of the immune system. The most common serotype, HIV-1, is distributed worldwide, while HIV-2 is primarily confined to West Africa.

IL-6

A gene on chromosome 7p21 that encodes interleukin-6, a cytokine which plays a role in the acute-phase response of inflammation and in B-cell maturation. It is primarily produced at sites of acute and chronic inflammation, where it is secreted into the serum and induces a transcriptional inflammatory response through Il-6 receptor alpha.

Interferon-γ:

A family of glycoprotein biological response modifiers used as antineoplastic agents and immunoregulators; they inhibit cellular growth, alter the state of cellular differentiation, have effects on the cell cycle, interfere with oncogene expression, alter cell surface antigen expression, have effects on antibody production, and regulate cytotoxic effector cells.

Kaposi's Sarcoma (KS):

A cancer characterized by numerous bluish-red nodules on the skin, usually on the lower extremities, that is endemic to equatorial Africa and often occurs in a particularly virulent form in people with AIDS.

Lymphadenopathy-Associated Virus (LAV):

A human T-cell lymphotropic virus type III; a cytopathic retrovirus (genus *Lentvirus*, family *Retroviridae*) that is 100-120 nm in diameter, has a lipid envelope, and has a characteristic dense cylindric nucleoid containing core proteins and genomic RNA.

Leukoencephalopathy:

Any of a group of diseases affecting the white substance of the brain. The term leukodystrophy is used to denote such disorders due to defective formation and maintenance of myelin in infants and children.

Lipodystrophy Syndrome:

A side effect encountered in the treatment of HIV patients with protease inhibitors in which they develop abnormal accumulations of body fat (e.g., over the upper back), hypercholesterolemia, hyperglycemia, hypertriglyceridemia, and insulin resistance.

Long-Term Survivors:

Persons who have experienced prolonged survival of HIV infection. This includes the full spectrum of untreated, HIV-infected long-term asymptomatic to those with AIDS who have survived due to successful treatment.

Lymphadenopathy:

A systemic disorder resembling lymphoma characterized by fever, night sweats, weight loss, generalized lymphadenopathy, hepatosplenomegaly, macropapular rash, polyclonal hypergammaglobulinemia, and Coombs'-positive hemolytic anemia.

Macrophages:

White blood cells whose job is to destroy invading microorganisms. *Listeria monocytogenes* avoids being killed and can multiply within the macrophage.

Maculopapular:

Pertaining to a cutaneous eruption consisting of both macules and papules.

Major Histocompatibility (MHC):

The quality of a cellular or tissue graft enabling it to be accepted and functional when transplanted to another organism.

Menigitus:

Meningitis is a serious inflammation of the meninges, the thin, membranous covering of the brain and the spinal cord. Meningitis is most commonly caused by infection (by bacteria, viruses, or fungi), although it can also be caused by bleeding into the meninges, cancer, diseases of the immune system, and an inflammatory response to certain types of chemotherapy or other chemical agents.

Monocytes:

The largest of the white blood cells. They have one nucleus and a large amount of grayish-blue cytoplasm. Develop into macrophages and both consume foreign material and alert T cells to its presence.

Monoclonal Antibodies:

Antibodies (immunoglobulins) produced by hybrid B lymphocyte tumors (myelomas). The type of antibodies produced depend on the selection of the B cell. These can be fused to cultured mouse, or even human, myeloma cells to form immortal tumours (hybridomas)-clones of cells that continue indefinitely to generate large quantities of the particular antibody produced by the B cell.

Mononucleosis:

An acute infectious disease that causes changes in the leukocytes; it is caused by the Epstein-Barr virus and is usually transmitted by direct oral contact (which is why it is sometimes called the "kissing disease"). It occurs more frequently in the spring and affects primarily children and young adults.

Mycobacterium Avium Complex:

A genus of gram-positive, aerobic, acid-fast bacteria, occurring as slightly curved or straight rods. It contains many species, including the highly pathogenic organisms that cause tuberculosis.

Mycobacterium Tuberculosis (TB):

Tuberculosis (TB) is a potentially fatal contagious disease that can affect almost any part of the body but is an infection of the lungs. It is caused by a bacterial microorganism, the tubercle bacillus or Mycobacterium tuberculosis.

Neuropathy:

Any of numerous functional disturbances and pathologic changes in the peripheral nervous system. The etiology may be known (e.g., arsenical, diabetic, ischemic, or traumatic neuropathy) or unknown. Encephalopathy and myelopathy are corresponding terms relating to involvement of the brain and spinal cord.

Nucleic Acid Testing (NAT):

Any of a group of long, linear macromolecules, either DNA or various types of RNA, that carry genetic information directing all cellular functions: composed of linked nucleotides.

Neuroendocrine Peptides:

Of, relating to, or involving the interaction between the nervous system and the hormones of the endocrine glands.

Nonnucleoside Reverse Transcriptase Inhibitors (NNRTIs):

A class of antiretroviral drugs that inhibit human immunodeficiency virus replication by blocking the reverse transcriptase enzyme essential for viral replication. These drugs have a different mechanism of action and side-effect profile from other reverse transcriptase inhibitors.

Pentamidine:

A drug used in the treatment of Pneumocystis Carinii Pneumonia and Trypanosomiasis. It was the exceptional demand for pentamidine in 1981 that heralded the onset of the AIDS pandemic. The drug is on the WHO official list.

Pneumocystis pneumonia:

An acute or chronic disease marked by inflammation of the lungs, usually caused by a bacterium, virus, or other infectious agent.

Progressive Lumbosacral Polyradiculopathy:

Progressive polyradiculopathy typically occurs late in the course of HIV infection, unlike inflammatory demyelinating polyradiculoneuropathies in HIV, which usually occur earlier in the course of disease. Progressive polyradiculopathy in HIV is extremely uncommon, however, is more prevalent in untreated patients with severe immunosuppression. Given its rare occurrence, incidence rate is unknown. HIV-infected patients become susceptible to progressive polyradiculopathy in advanced immunosuppression when the CD4 T-cell count is less than 50/µL.

Progressive Multifocal Leukoencephalopathy (PML):

PML is a rapidly progressive neuromuscular disease caused by opportunistic infection of brain cells (oligodendrocytes and astrocytes) by the JC virus (JCV).

Seropositive:

Indicating a positive reaction to a serological blood test, especially one testing for the presence of antibodies.

Simian immunodeficiency virus (SIV):

Any of several strains of a retrovirus of the genus *Lentivirus* that cause an immunodeficiency syndrome similar to AIDS in primates by infecting helper T cells of the immune system.

Spastic Paraparesis:

A partial paralysis of the lower extremities.

Tardive Dyskinesia (TD):

Tardive dyskinesia is a mostly irreversible neurological disorder of involuntary movements caused by long-term use of antipsychotic or neuroleptic drugs.

T-Lymphocytes:

A lymphocyte formed in the bone marrow from which it migrates to the thymic cortex to become an immunologically competent cell; T lymphocytes have long lifespans (months to years) and are responsible for cell-mediated immunity; T lymphocytes form rosettes with sheep erythrocytes and differentiate and divide in the presence of transforming agents (mitogens); T lymphocytes have characteristic T cell receptor-CD3 complexes as surface markers and may be further categorized by function, such as helper and cytotoxic.

Toxoplasma Gondii:

A species of obligate intracellular coccidian protozoans which has its sexual cycle in the GI tract of its definitive host.

Trichomoniasis:

Trichomoniasis refers to an infection of the genital and urinary tract. It is the most common sexually transmitted disease, affecting about 120 million women worldwide each year.

Tumor Necrosis Factor (TNF-a):

TNF-a is a pro-inflammatory cytokine that is released by glial cells and acts on neurons through its receptor TNFR1.

DRUGS

3TC - (Lamivudine):

3TC is a well-tolerated cytidine analog. Rapid development of resistance, and only one-point mutation (M184V) is required, which, however, increases the sensitivity of AZT-resistant viruses and reduces viral fitness. 3TC is also effective against hepatitis B virus.

Abacavir - (ABC):

An antiviral drug, $C_{14}H_{18}N_6O$, that is a nucleoside reverse transcriptor inhibitor and is used in its sulfate form in combination with other drugs for the treatment of HIV infection.

Acyclovir - (Zovirax):

An antiretroviral medication used for the treatment and prophylaxis of HSV and VZV infections.

A relatively well-tolerated PI, which can be given once daily. It has a favorable lipid profile in comparison to other PIs. The most common side effects are elevated bilirubin levels, which not unusually manifest as jaundice.

Amprenavir:

A protease inhibitor used with other antiretrovirals for managing HIV-1 (e.g., nelfinavir, indinavir or saquinavir).

Amyl Nitrate:

A volatile yellow liquid, $C_5H_{11}NO_2$, formerly used in medicine as a vasodilator, but now replaced by other nitrates, such as nitroglycerin. It is used illicitly to induce euphoria and enhance sexual stimulation.

Aripiprazole:

Aripiprazole is used to treat the symptoms of schizophrenia (a mental illness that causes disturbed or unusual thinking, loss of interest in life, and strong or inappropriate emotions) in adults and teenagers 13 years of age and older.

Atripla:

Atripla is the first complete HAART in a single combination tablet (300 mg tenofovir, 200 mg emtricitabin and 600 mg efavirenz), which in addition, only needs to be taken once daily.

AZT - (Zidovudine):

AZT is a thymidine analog, and the oldest HIV drug, and continues to be a component of many HAART regimens and transmission prophylaxis. It has good CNS penetration. The most common side effect is myelotoxicity which may cause severe anemia. Unfortunately, once daily dosing is not possible.

Buspirone:

Buspirone is a prescription medication used to treat anxiety. It belongs to a group of anti-anxiety drugs called anxiolytics, but it seems to work somewhat differently than other drugs in the class.

Chlorpromazine:

A phenothiazine used in the form of the base or the hydrochloride salt as an antipsychotic agent, antiemetic, and presurgical sedative, and in the treatment of intractable hiccups, acute intermittent porphyria, tetanus, and the manic phase of bipolar disorder. It is also used to treat certain severe behavioral problems in children.

Clindamycin:

A semisynthetic antibiotic that is a derivative of Lincomycin and is used to treat gram-positive penicillin-resistant infections. Destroys gram-negative bacteria by irreversibly binding to 30S subunit of bacterial ribosomes and blocking protein synthesis, resulting in misreading of genetic code and separation of ribosomes from messenger RNA.

Clonidine:

A centrally acting antihypertensive agent, administered orally as the hydrochloride salt; also used to treat migraine, dysmenorrhea, opioid withdrawal, vasomotor symptoms of menopause, and cancer-associated pain.

Combivir:

In cases of reduced renal function (creatinine clearance below 50 ml/min) and anemia, Combivir should be replaced with the individual drugs to allow for adjustment of 3TC and AZT doses.

Darunivir:

Inhibits HIV-1 protease, selectively inhibiting the cleavage of HIV-encoded specific polyproteins in infected cells. This prevents the formation of mature virus particles.

d4T - (Stavudine):

Stavudine is a thymidine analog. Subjective tolerability is good, and the drug was long considered an important alternative to AZT. Due to the mitochondrial toxicity (lipoatrophy, lactic acidosis, peripheral neuropathy), particularly in combination with ddI, the (long-term) use of d4T is not recommended.

TMC-114 - (Darunavir):

Darunavir is a new, well-tolerated PI with considerable activity against PI-resistant viruses and was recently licensed in Europe and the USA. Darunavir can be boosted with ritonavir.

Desipramine:

A tricyclic antidepressant of the dibenzazepine group, administered orally as the hydrochloride salt.

ddI - (Didanosine):

ddI was one of the first NRTIs, which today, because of its side effects (pancreatitis 10 %) and mitochondrial toxicity, is only used in certain resistance situations. The dose has to be adjusted according to body weight.

Delavirdine:

Delavirdine is rarely used today, due to high dosing and drug interactions.

Diazepam:

Diazepam is a benzodiazepine. It affects chemicals in the brain that may be unbalanced in people with anxiety. It is used to treat anxiety disorders, alcohol withdrawal symptoms, or muscle spasms.

Dolutegravir:

Treatment of HIV-1 infection, in combination with other antiretrovirals.

Efavirenz:

Efavirenz is a frequently used NNRTI. The diverse CNS side effects are a substantial problem (disturbances of sleep architecture, morning dizziness, somnolence). Further disadvantages include drug interactions, and cross-resistance, as with the other members of this drug class.

Elvitegravir:

Treatment of HIV-1 infection, in combination with a protease inhibitor plus ritonavir and other antiretrovirals in treatment-experienced adults.

Emtricitabine - (FTC):

Emtricitabine is a well-tolerated cytidine analog, comparable to 3TC, and both biochemically have the same resistance profile, but has a longer half-life Retrieved from *https://medical-dictionary.thefreedictionary.com/*

Etravirin - (TMC-125):

Etravirin is a NNRTI, which is also effective against NNRTI-resistant HIV strains. Since February 2007, etravirin has been available in an Expanded Access Program.

Fluconazole:

Fluconazole is an antifungal azole, and the drug of choice for treatment of candidiasis in HIV infection and for secondary prophylaxis of cryptococcosis. It is also a component of acute therapy for cryptococcosis.

Fosamprenavir:

Fosamprenavir is a calcium phosphate ester of amprenavir, which is more soluble, and is better absorbed than amprenavir. The overall tolerability is fairly good.

Foscarnet:

An agent that inhibits replication of viruses, used as the sodium salt in treatment of cytomegalovirus retinitis and herpes simplex in immune compromised patients.

Gancyclavir:

A derivative of Acylovir used in the form of the base or the sodium salt in treatment of cytomegalovirus.

Gp 120:

A glycoprotein that protrudes from the surface of the HIV virus and binds to the glycoprotein CD4 in human cells.

Indinavir:

Indinavir was, in 1996, one of the first PIs. However today, its use is limited due to side effects, especially skin and renal problems.

Lamotrigine:

An anticonvulsive used in treatment of certain forms of epilepsy.

Lithium:

Lithium is used to treat and prevent episodes of mania (frenzied, abnormally excited mood) in people with bipolar disorder (manic-depressive disorder; a disease that causes episodes of depression, episodes of mania, and other abnormal moods).

Lopinavir:

An effective PI in treatment-naïve patients, as well as treatment-experienced patients. Disadvantages include gastrointestinal side effects (diarrhea) and the often-significant dyslipidemia, which is more extreme than with some other PIs. As with all PIs, lipodystrophy and various drug interactions should be considered.

Lorazapam:

Lorazepam is the generic form of the brand-name drug Ativan, used to treat anxiety disorders and to relieve anxiety that's associated with depression. Lorazepam is also used to treat insomnia

Maraviroc:

HIV infection (with other antiretrovirals), specifically in treatment-experienced or treatment-naive patients with CCR5–tropic HIV-1 infection. Genetic Implication Use should be determined by tropism testing.

Metoclorpromide:

A dopamine receptor antagonist and prokinetic agent that stimulates gastric motility, used as the hydrochloride salt as an antiemetic, an aid in gastrointestinal radiology and intestinal intubaion, and in treatment of gastroparesis and gastroesophageal reflux; administered orally, intravenously, or intramuscularly.

Nelfinavir:

Nelfinavir is a well-tolerated PI but is slightly less potent than boosted PIs.

Neostigmine Methylsulfate:

A Non-nucleoside reverse transcriptase inhibitor. Muscle stimulant.

Nevirapine:

Nevirapine is a frequently prescribed NNRTI, which is also used successfully for the prevention of mother-to-child transmission. As with all NNRTIs, a single point mutation is sufficient to develop high-level resistance. It has a very good long-term tolerability, also has a favorable lipid profile), hepatotoxicity within the first months of treatment is a problem.

Olanzapine:

A monoaminergic antagonist used as an antipsychotic agent; administered orally.

Pentamidine:

An antiinfective used as the isethionate salt, administered intravenously or intramuscularly in treatment of early African Trypanosomiasis and Leishmaniasis and intravenously, intramuscularly, or by oral inhalation in treatment and prophylaxis of *Pneumocystis carinii*.

Pyrimethamine:

A folic acid antagonist used as an antimalarial agent, especially for suppressive prophylaxis, and also used concomitantly with a sulphonamide in treatment of toxoplasmosis.

Quetiapine:

Quetiapine is an antipsychotic medicine. It works by changing the actions of chemicals in the brain. Quetiapine is used to treat schizophrenia in adults and children who are at least 13 years old.

Raltegravir - (MK-0518):

Raltegravir is an integrase inhibitor, that was made available in 2007 through an expanded-access program for patients with viruses that are resistant to at least one of the drug classes: NRTIs, NNRTIs and PIs. This drug is well tolerated and has a promising drug in therapy-naive as well as treatment -experienced patients.

Risperidone:

Risperidone is an antipsychotic medicine that works by changing the effects of chemicals in the brain. Risperidone is used to treat schizophrenia in adults and children who are at least 13 years old.

Ritonavir:

Due to its gastrointestinal side effects, the therapeutic dose of ritonavir is rarely prescribed, however, at lower doses it is frequently used for boosting and is better tolerated. It also has numerous interactions.

Saquinavir:

Saquinavir was the first PI to be licensed for HIV therapy in 1995. Apart from gastrointestinal problems, saquinavir is well tolerated. Today, it is only used boosted with ritonavir. Since the introduction of the 500-mg capsule, the number of tablets taken has been significantly reduced.

Sodenosyl Methoionine (SAM-E):

A sulfur-containing amino acid, one of the essential amino acids, furnishing both methyl groups and sulfur necessary for metabolism.

Sulfadiazine:

One of a group of diazine derivatives of sulfanilamide, the pyrimidine analogue of sulfapyridine, and sulfathiazole; one of the components of the triple sulfonamide mixture. It is an inhibitor of bacterial folic acid synthesis, which has been highly effective against pneumococcal, staphylococcal, and streptococcal infections, against infections with *Escherichia coli* and *Klebsiella pneumoniae*, and in acute gonococcal arthritis; sulfadiazine sodium has the same uses.

Sulfonomide:

A class of organic compounds that are amides of sulphonic acids, some of which are sulpha drugs and act as powerful inhibitors of bacterial activity, although bacteria have become increasingly resistant to them. Examples are sulphadimidine and sulphadiazine.

Tenofovir:

Tenofovir DF is the prodrug of the acyclic nucleotide analog tenofovir, and has good oral bioavailability, and is well tolerated, and low mitochondrial toxicity, however, potential nephrotoxicity and a few interactions must be considered (ddI, atazanavir). It also has a good efficacy in fighting the hepatitis B virus.

Tetravalent:

Chemistry: having valence 4. Immunology: having four sites of attachment. Used of an antibody or antigen. Containing antigens from four strains of a microorganism or virus. Used of a vaccine or serum.

Tipranavir:

Tipranavir is the first nonpeptidic protease inhibitor (PI), which was superior to other boosted PIs in two large studies on intensively PI-treatment-experienced patients. Important salvage drug, and moderately hepatotoxic, and has to be boosted with increased ritonavir doses.

Trizivir:

The combination AZT+3TC+abacavir is virologically not as effective as "divergent: combinations, and today is only an option for patients with compliance problems, and with co-medications that have many interactions (tuberculostatics). In addition to further disadvantages, it causes mitochondrial toxicity.

Truvada:

Truvada is a much-used combination preparation, containing tenofovir and emtricitabine. Overall, it is very tolerable, but close monitoring of renal function is needed.

Tybost:

To increase blood levels of atazanivir and darunavir (in combination with other antiretrovirals) in the treatment of HIV-1 infection.

Valganciclovir:

Valganciclovir is the first CMV drug with good efficacy that can be administered orally, and to a large extent overshadows all other substances. Valganciclovir is a prodrug of ganciclovir, and therefore has a similar toxicity profile.

Venlafaxline:

Venlafaxine is used to treat depression. It may improve your mood and energy level, and may help restore your interest in daily living. Venlafaxine is known as a serotonin-norepinephrine ...

Voriconazole:

Voriconazole is an orally available azole antimycotic, which is the therapy of choice for invasive aspergillosis. It is also active against invasive Candida infections.

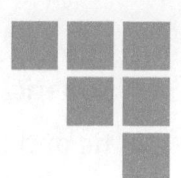

REFERENCES

Aberg, J.A. (2012). Aging, inflammation, and HIV infection. Topics in Antiviral Medicine, 20,101-105.

AIDS: the Early Years and CDC's Response (2011). Retrieved from https://www.cdc.gov/mmwr/preview/mmwrhtml/su6004a11.htm

Althoff, KN. Gange, SJ. Klein, MB. et al. (2010). Late presentation for human immunodeficiency virus care in the United States and Canada. Clin Infect Dis.; 50 (11):1512-1520. Available at: http://www.ncbi.nlm.nih.gov/pubmed/20415573

American Academy of HIV Medicine. (2007). Pain Management. In: AAHIVM Fundamentals of HIV Medicine (2007 ed.). Washington, DC: American Academy of HIV Medicine

American Psychiatric Association: (1994). Diagnostic and Statistical Manual of Mental Disorders, 4th ed (DSM-IV). Washington, DC, APA, [F]

Ammann, AJ. Cowan, MJ. Wara, DW. et al. (1983). Acquired immunodeficiency in an infant: possible transmission by means of blood products. Lancet 1: 956-8. http://amedeo.com/lit.php?id=6132270

Angelino, AF. Treisman, GJ. (2001). Management of psychiatric disorders in patients infected with human immunodeficiency virus, Clin Infect Dis, vol. 33 (pg. 847-56)

Antiretroviral HIV Drugs: Side Effects & Adherence Healthline (2017) Retrieved fromhttps://www.healthline.com/health/hiv-aids/antiretroviral-drugs-side-effects-adherence

Amsalu, Belete. Gashaw, Andaregie. Minale, Tareke. Tigabu, Birhan. Telake, Azale. (2014). Prevalence of Anxiety and Associated Factors among People Living with HIV/AIDS at Debretabor General Hospital Anti Retro Viral Clinic

Atkinson, JH Jr. Grant, I. Kennedy, CJ. Richman, DD. Spector, SA. McCutchan, JA. (1988). Prevalence of psychiatric disorders among men infected with human immunodeficiency virus: a controlled study. Arch Gen Psychiatry, vol. 45 (pg. 859-64)

Baastrup, PC. Schou, M. (1983). Lithium as a prophylactic agent: its effect against recurrent depressions and manic-depressive psychosis, Arch Gen Psychiatry, 1967, vol. 16 (pg. 162-72)

Barre-Sinoussi, F. Chermann, JC. Rey. et al. Isolation of a T-lymphotropic retrovirus from a patient at risk for AIDS. Science 220: 868-71. http://amedeo.com/lit.php?id=6189183

Barre-Sinoussi, F. Chermann, JC. Rey, F. at al. Isolation of a T-lymphotropic retrovirus from a patient at risk for acquired immune deficiency syndrome (AIDS) Science 1983;220:868-71. [PubMed]

Bayer, R. (1989). Private Acts, Social Consequences: AIDS and the Politics of Public Health. New York: The FreePress, 1. (p. 24)

Bayer, R. Oppenheimer, G. AIDS Doctors: (2000). Voices from the Epidemic. New York: Oxford University Press

Bhatia, R. Ryscavage, P. and Taiwo, B. (2012). Accelerated aging and human Immunodeficiency virus infection: Emerging challenges of growing older in the era of successful antiretroviral therapy. Journal of Neurovirology, 18, 247-55. doi: 10.1007/s13365-011-0073-y. Epub 2011 Dec 29.

Bhavan, KP. Kampalath, VN. Overton ET. (2008). The aging of the HIV epidemic.

CDC. (1982). Possible transfusion-associated acquired immune deficiency syndrome (AIDS)---California. MMWR 31:652-4.

Bing, EG. Burnam, MA. Longshore, D. (2001). Psychiatric disorders and drug use among human immunodeficiency virus-infected adults in the United States, Arch Gen Psychiatry, vol. 58 (pg. 721-8)

Blessing, Gelln J. Forister, Dennis J. (2015). Introduction to Research and Medical Literature for Health Professionals 4th Edition, Jones and Bartlett

Bornstein, RA. Nasrallah, HA. Para M.F et al. (1991), Rate of CD4 decline and neuropsychological performance in HIV infection. Arch Neurol 48(7):704-707.

Cameron, DW. Japour, AJ. Xu, Y. et al. (1999). Ritonavir and saquinavir combination therapy for the treatment of HIV infection. AIDS 13: 213-24. http://amedeo.com/lit.php?id=10202827

Carey, MP. Carey, KB. Maisto, SA. et al. (2004), HIV risk behavior among psychiatric outpatients: association with psychiatric disorder, substance use disorder, and gender. J Nerv Ment Dis 192(4):289-296

Carr, A. Workman, C, Smith, DE. et al. (2002). Abacavir substitution for nucleoside analogs in patients with HIV lipoatrophy: a randomized trial. JA MA 288: 207-15. http://a medeo.com/lit.php?id=12095385

CD4 T Luymphocyte | Definition | AIDSinfo (2017). Retrieved from https://aidsinfo.nih.gov/understanding-hiv-aids/glossary/113/cd4-t-lymphocyte

CDC. Kaposi's sarcoma and Pneumocystis pneumonia among homosexual men (1981). New York City and California. MMWR; 30:305-308

CDC. Pneumocystis pneumonia (1981). Los Angeles. MMWR 1; 30:250–252. Centers for Disease Control and Prevention. (2008). HIV/AIDS among persons age 50 and older. Retrieved from http://www.cdc.gov/hiv/az.htm.

CDC. (1982). Possible transfusion-associated acquired immune deficiency syndrome (AIDS)---California. MMWR 31:652-4.

CDC. Revision of the case definition of acquired immunodeficiency syndrome for national reporting—United States. MMWR 1985:34:373-5. [PubMed]

Centers for Disease Control Task force on Kaposi's Sarcoma and Opportunistic Infections. (1982). Epidemiologic aspects of the current outbreak of Kaposi's sarcoma and opportunistic infections. N Engl J Med; 302:

Cherner, M. Ellis, R. Lazzaretto, D. (2004). Effects of HIV-1 infection and aging on neurobehavioral functioning: preliminary findings. AIDS.;18 (suppl1): S27-S34 [PubMed]

Clavel, F. Guetard, D. Brun-Vezinet, F. Chamaret, S. Rey, MA. (1986). Santos-Ferreira, O. Isolation of a new human retrovirus from West African patients with AIDS. Science 233: 343

Cohen, MS. Chen, YQ. McCauley, M. et al. (2016). Antiretroviral therapy for the prevention of HIV-1 transmission. N Engl J Med. 375(9):830-839. Available at: https://www.ncbi.nlm.nih.gov/pubmed/27424812

Comorbidities: (2012). A concomitant but unrelated pathologic or disease process; usually used in epidemiology to indicate the coexistence of two or more disease processes. Farlex Partner Medical Dictionary. Retrieved from https://medical-dictionary.thefreedictionary.com/Comorbiditirs

Confalonieri, M. Calderini, E. Terraciano, S. et al (2002). Non-invasive ventilation for treating acute respiratory failure in AIDS patients with Pneumocystis carinii pneumonia. Intensive Care Med 28:1233-8 http://amedeo.com/lit.php?id=12209270

Connick, E. (2005). Incomplete antibody evolution and seoreversion after treatment of primary HIV type 1 infection: What is the clinical significance? Clin Infect Dis 40:874ñ5. http://amedeo.com/lit.php?id=15736022

Cooper, D. Gold, J. Maclean, P. et al. (1985). Acute AIDS retrovirus infection. Definition of a clinical illness associated with seroconversion. Lancet 1:537-540. http://amedeo.com/lit.php?id=28578997

Corral, I. Quereda, C, Garcia-Villanueva, M et al (2004). Focalmonophasic demyelinating leukoencephalopathy in advanced HIV infection.

Eur Neurol; 52 (1): 36-41 [PubMed]

Curr, L. HIV/AIDS Rep.; 5 (3):150-158 [PubMed]

Dalakas, MC. Illa, I. Pezeshkpour, GH. Laukaitis, JP. Cohen, B. & Griffin, JL. (1990). Mitochondrial myopathy caused by long-term zidovudine therapy. New England Journal of Medicine, 322(16):1098-105.

Dalgleish, AG. Beverley, PC. Clapham, PR. et al (1984). The CD4 (T4) antigen is an essential component of the receptor for the AIDS retrovirus. Nature 312: 763-7. http://amedeo.com/lit.php?id=6096719

Dannemann, B. McCutchan, JA. Israelski, D. et al (1992). Treatment of toxoplasmic encephalitis in patients with AIDS. A randomized trial comparing pyrimethamine plus clindamycin to pyrimethamine plus sulfadiazine. Ann Intern Med 116:3 3-43. http://amedeo.com/lit.php?id=1727093

Debretabor, Amhara. Ethiopia, (2014). *American Journal of Psychiatry and Neuroscience.* Vol. 2, No. 6, 2014, pp. 109-114. doi: 10.11648/j.ajpn.20140206.15

Deeks, SG. (2010). HIV infection, inflammation, immunosenescence, and aging. Annu Rev Med.; 62:141–155.

[PMC free article] [PubMed] DNA vs RNA (1981). Difference and Comparison I Differn Retrieved from https://www.diffen.com › Science › Biology › Microbiology

Dilley, JW. Ochitill, HN. Perl M. Volberding, PA. (1985). Findings in psychiatric consultations with patients with acquired immunodeficiency syndrome. Am J Psychiatry 142(1):82-86

Dolder, CR. Patterson, TL. Jeste, DV. (2004). HIV, psychosis and aging: past, present and future. AIDS. 18(Suppl 1): S35-S42. [PubMed]

Durack, DT. (2017). Opportunistic infections and Kaposi's sarcoma in homosexual men. N Engl J Med; 305:1465-1467

Effros, RB. Fletcher, CV. Gebo, K. et al (2008). Aging and infectious diseases: workshop on HIV infection and aging: what is known and future research directions. Clin Infect Dis.; 47(4): 542-553 [PMC free article] [PubMed]

Ellis, RJ. Badiee, J. Vaida, F. Letendre, S. Heaton, RK. Clifford, D. Collier, AC. Gelman, B. McArthur, J. Morgello, S. McCutchan, JA. Grant, I. (2011). CD4 nadir is a predictor of HIV neurocognitive impairment in the era of combination antiretroviral therapy. AIDS.; 25:1747-51. [PMC free article] [PubMed]

Evans, DL. Staab, JP. Petitto, JM. Morrison, MF. Szuba, MP. Ward, HE. et al (1999). Depression in the medical setting: biopsychological interactions and treatment considerations. J Clin Psychiatry 60 (Suppl 4):40-55. [PubMed]

Fanning, Rachlis A. (1993). MM. Zidovudine toxicity. Clinical features and management. Drug Safety 8:312-320

Farber, EW. Mc Daniel, JS. (2002). Clinical management of psychiatric disorders in patients with HIV disease. Psychiatr Q 73: 5-16 http://amedeo.com/lit.php?id=11780597

Ferrando, S. van Gorp, W. McElhiney, M. et al (1998), Highly active antiretroviral treatment in HIV infection: benefits for neuropsychological function. AIDS 12(8): F65-F70

Fischl, MA. Richman, DD. Grieco, MH. et al (1987). The efficacy of azidothymidine (AZT) in the treatment of patients with AIDS and AIDS-related complex. A double-blind, placebo-controlled trial. N Engl J Med 317185–191.

Forstein, M. (1984). The psychosocial impact of the acquired immunodeficiency syndrome. Semin Oncol 11(1):77-82.

Foster, R. Olajide, D. Everall, I. (2003). Antiretroviral therapy-induced psychosis: case report and brief review of the literature. HIV Med 4:139-44. http://amedeo.com/lit.php?id=12702135

Franceschini, N. Napravnik, S. Eron, JJ Jr, et al. (2005). Incidence and etiology of acute renal failure among ambulatory HIV-infected patients. Kidney Int. Apr; 67(4):1526-31.

Gallo, RC. Essex, M. Gross, L. (1984). Human T-Cell Leukemia-Lymphoma Virus: The Family of Human T-Lymphotropic Retroviruses-Their Role In Malignancies And Association With AIDS. New York, Cold Spring Harbor Press

Gallo, RC. Salahuddin, SZ. Popovic, M. et al. (1984). Frequent detection and isolation of cytopathic retroviruses (HTLV-III) from patients with AIDS and at risk for AIDS. Science 224:500-3. [PubMed]

Global AIDS Update (2016). - unaids Retrieved from https://www.hiv.gov/hiv-basics/overview/data-and-trends/global-statistics

Global Statisics I (2107). HIV.gov Retrieved from http://www.unaids.org/sites/default/files/media_asset/global-AIDS-update-2016_en.pdf

Goethe, KE. Mitchell, JE. Marshall, DW. et al. (1989). Neuropsychological and neurological function of human immunodeficiency virus seropositive asymptomatic individuals. Arch Neurol 46(2):129-133.

Gonzalez, A. Zvolensky, MJ. Parent, J. Grover, KW. Hickey, M. (2012). HIV symptom distress and anxiety sensitivity in relation to panic, social anxiety, and depression symptoms among HIV-positive adults. AIDS Patient Care and STDs (epub) (Jan 16)

Gottlieb, MS. Schroff, R. Schanker, HM. et al (1981). Pneumocystis carinii pneumonia and mucosal candidiasis inpreviously healthy homosexual men: evidence of a new acquired cellular immunodeficiency. N Engl J Med; 305:1425–1431

Grabar, S. Kousignian, I. Sobel, A. Le Bras, P. Gasnault, J. Enel, P. Jung, C. Mahamat, A Lang, JM Costagliola, D (2004). Immunologic and clinical responses to highly active antiretroviral therapy over 50 years of age. Results from the French Database on HIV. AIDS.18:2029-2038. [PubMed]

Green, WC. (1991). The molecular biology of HIV-1 infection. New England Journal of Medicine, 324: 308-16

Grimes, DA. Schulz, KF. (2002). Cohort studies: marching towards outcomes. The Lancet, volume 359, pages 341-345

Hall, CD Snyder, CR Messenheimer, JA Wilkins, J. Robertson, WT Whaley, RA & Robertson, KR. (1991). Peripheral neuropathy in a cohort of human immunodeficiency virus-infected patients. Incidence and relationship to other nervous system dysfunction. Archives of Neurology, 48(12): 1273-4

Halstead, S. Riccio, Harlow. P, Oretti R. Thompson, C. (1988) Psychosis Associated with HIV Infection. Br J Psychiatry 153: 618-623

Haverkos, HW. Gottlieb, MS. Killen, JY. Edelman, R. Classification of HTLV-III/LAV-related diseases [Letter] J Infect Dis 1985;152:1095. [PubMed]

Havlik, R.J. Karpiak, M. Cantor, M. H. & Shippy, R A. (2009). Health status, comorbidities, and health-related quality of life. In: Brennan, (Eds.). Research on older adults with HIV: An in-depth examination of an emerging population. New York: Nova Science, pp.

Marzolini, C. Telenti, A. Decosterd, LA. et al. (2001). Efavirenz plasma levels can predict treatment failure and central nervous system side effects in HIV-1-infected patients. AIDS 15:71-75. http://amedeo.com/lit.php?id=11192870

Heimer, R. Myers, SS. Cadman, EC. et al. (1992). Detection by polymerase chain reaction of human immunodeficiency virus type 1 proviral DNA sequences in needles of injecting drug users. J Infect Dis 165:781.

Himmelhoch, S. Medoff, DR. (2002). Efficacy of antidepressant medication among HIV-positive individuals with depression: a systematic review and meta-analysis. AIDS Patient Care STDS 19:813-22 http://amedeo.com/lit.php?id=16375613 HIV Drugs and the HIV Lifecycle The Well Project (2017). Retrieved from http:www.thewellproject.org/hiv-infor-mation/hiv-drugs-and-hiv-lifecycle

HIV neurocognitive impairment in the era of combination antiretroviral therapy. (2017). AIDS.; 25:1747-51. [PMC free article] [PubMed]

HIV/AIDS Information (2017). Retrieved from https://dhhr.wv.gov/oeps/std-hiv-hep/HIV_AIDSInformation.aspx

HIV.gov retrieved from https://www.hiv.gov/hiv-basics/overview/history/hiv-and-aids-timeline

Holland, JC. Tross, S. (1985). The psychosocial and neuropsychiatric sequelae of the acquired immunodeficiency syndrome and related disorders. Ann Intern Med 103(5):760-764

Ho, DD. Neumann, AU. Perelson, AS. Chen, W. Leonard, JM. Markowitz, M. (1995). Rapid turnover of plasma virions and CD4 lymphocytes in HIV-1 infection. Nature 373:123-6. http://amedeo.com/lit.php?id=7816094

Holtzman, DM. Kaku, DA. So, YT. (1989). New-onset seizures associated with human immunodeficiency virus infection: causation and clinical features in 100 cases. Am J Med. Aug; 87(2):173-7 [PubMed ID: 2757058]

How to Choose from the Different Research Methods (2017). Retrieved from http://www.home.cc.gatech.edu/cmgardne/.../Research%20Methods%20and%20Designs. docx.pdf Journal of Acquired Immune Deficiency Syndrome, 31(2): 171-7

How to Manage Your HIV Pain (n.d.). Healthline Retrieved from http://www.healthline.com/health/hiv-aids/managing-pain

HRSA HIV-Associated Dementia and Other Neuro-cognitive Disorders. (2014). Guide for HIV/AIDS

Kahn, JO. Walker, BD. Acute human immunodeficiency virus type 1 infection. (1998). New England Journal of Medicine 339:33-39

Kalayjian, RC. Al-Harthi, L. (2009). HIV and the Brain: New Challenges in the Modern Era: The Effects of Aging on HIV Disease. 1st ed. New York, NY: Humana Press:331-347

Kaufmann, DE. Lichterfeld, M. Altfeld, M. et al (2004). Limited Durability of Viral Control following Treated Acute HIV Infection. PLOS Medicine in press http://www.plosmedicine.org/perslev/?request=get-document&doi=10.1371/journal.pmed.0010036

Kirk, O. Mocroft, A. Katzenstein, TL. et al (1998). Changes in use of antiretroviral therapy in regions of Europe over time. AIDS12: 2031-9. http://amedeo.com/lit.php?id=9814872

Koppel, BS. Wormser, GP. Tuchman, AJ. Maayan, S. Hewlett, D. Jr & Daras, M. (1985). Central nervous system involvement in patients with acquired immune deficiency syndrome (AIDS). Acta Neuro-logy Scandinavica, 71(5):337-53

Koralnik, IJ. Beaumanoir, A. Hausler, R. et al (1990). A controlled study of early neurologic abnormalities in men with asymptomatic human immunodeficiency virus infection. [Published erratum N Engl J Med 323(24):1716.] N Engl J Med 323(13):864-870 [see comment]

Koutsilieri, E. Scheller, I. Sopper, S. Meulen, V. ter and Riederer, P. (2002). Psychiatric complications in human immunodeficiency virus infection. Clinical Neurochemistry and NPF Center of Excellence Research Laboratory, Department of Psyc1hiatry and Psychotherapy and Institute of Virology and Immunobiology, University of Wuerzburg, Germany

Levy, JA. Hoffman, AD. Kramer, SM. Landis, JA. Shimabukuro, JM. Oshiro, LS. (1984). Isolation of lymphocytopathic retroviruses from San Francisco patients with AIDS. Science 225:840-2. [PubMed]

Levy, RM. Bredesen, DE. Rosenblum, ML. (1985). Neurological manifestations of the acquired immunodeficiency syndrome (AIDS): experience at UCSF and review of the literature. J Neurosurg. Apr; 62 (4):475-95 [PubMed ID: 2983051]

Liu, R. Paxton, WA. Choe, S. et al. (1996). Homozygous defect in HIV-1 coreceptor accounts for resistance of some multiply-exposed individuals to HIV-1 infection. Cell 86: 367-77. http://amedeo.com/lit.php?id=8756719

Lyketsos, CG. Hanson, AL. Fishman, M. Rosenblatt, A. McHugh, PR. & Treisman, GJ. (1993). Manic syndrome early and late in the course of HIV. American journal of Psychiatry 150:326-7

Mann, JM. Presentation at XII International Con-ference on AIDS, June 28-July 3, 1998, Geneva, Switzerland.

Marchioni, E. Tavazz, I E. Bono, G. et al. (2006). Headache attributed to infection: Observations on the HIS classification (ICHD-II). Cephalalgia.; 26:1427-1433

Marzani-Nissen, G. (2011). A pilot randomized clinical trial of two medication adherence and drug use interventions for HIV+ crack cocaine users. Drug Alcohol Depend. 116:177-187. Drug Alcohol Depend. 116:177-187. [PMC free article] [PubMed]

Martin, CP. Fain, MJ Klotz, SA. (2008). The older HIV-positive adult: a critical review of the medical literature. Am J Med;121:1032-1037. [PubMed]

Masur, H. Michelis, MA. Greene, JB. et al. (1981). An outbreak of community-acquired Pneumocystis carinii pneumonia: initial manifestation of cellular immune dysfunction. N Engl J Med 305:1431.

Maschke, M. Kastrup, O. Esser, S. et al. (2000). Incidence and prevalence of neurological disorders associated with HIV since the introduction of highly active antiretroviral therapy (HAART). J Neurol Neurosurg Psychiatry. Sep. 69 (3):376-80. [Medline]

McArthur, JC. Brew, BJ. (2010). HIV-associated neurocognitive disorders: is there a hidden epidemic? AIDS. 24:1367–1370. [PubMed]

McGuire, D. & Greene, WC. (1996). Neurological damage in HIV infection: The Molecular Biology of HIV/AIDS. New York: John Wiley & Sons,127-142

Medical Dictionary (2017). Retrieved from https://medical-dictionary.thefreedictionary.com/

Medical Definition of Antiprotozoal (2017). MedicineNet Retrieved from https://www.medicinenet.com/script/main/art.asp?articlekey=10216

EK, Bell J. (2010). Adherence to antiretroviral medications and medical care in HIV-infected adults diagnosed with mental and substance abuse disorders. AIDS Care.21:168-177. [PubMed]

Miller, EN. Selnes, OA. & McArthar, JC. (1990). Neuropsychological performance in HIV-1 infected homosexual men; the multicenter AIDS cohort study. Neurology, 40 197-203

Najera, R. Herrera, Ml. De Andres, R. (1987). Human immunodeficiency virus and related retroviruses, In

AIDS-A Global perspective [Special Issue]. West J Med 1 Dec; 147:702-708)

Nath, A, Berger, J (2004). HIV dementia. Current Treatment Options in Neurology 6(2):139-151

Neuenburg, JK. Brodt, HR. Herndier, BG. Bickel, M. Bacchetti, P. Price, RW. Grant, RM. & Schlote, W. (2002). HIV-related neuropathology, 1985 to 1999: rising prevalence of HIV encephalopathy in the era of highly active antiretroviral therapy. Journal of Acquired Immune Deficiency Syndrome, 31(2): 171-7

Neurologic and psychiatric complications of antiretroviral agents. – NCBI (2005). Retrieved from https://www.ncbi.nlm.nih.gov/pubmed/16433108 Neurological Complications of AIDS Fact Sheet (2017) National Institute of Retrieved from https://. ninds.nih.gov/.../Fact=Sheets/Neurological-Complications-AIDS-Fact-She...

Neuropsychiatric manifestations of HIV infection and AIDS (2005). Journal of Retrieved from http://www.jpn.ca/wp-content/uplaods/2014/30-4-237.pdf

Nichols, SE. (1985). Psychosocial reactions of persons with the acquired immunodeficiency syndrome. Ann Intern Med 103(5):765-767

Nguyen, N. Holodniy, M. (2008). HIV infection in the elderly. Clin Interv Aging.; 3:453-472. [PMC free article] [PubMed]

Oppenheimer, GM. (1988). In the Eye of the Storm: The Epidemiological Construction of AIDS. In: Fee E, Fox DM, editors. AIDS: The Burdens of History Berkeley, California: University of California Press; 1. pp. 267-300.

Ouagari, Z. Tubiana, R. Mohand, HA. et al. (2006). Skin rash associated with atazanavir: report of three cases. AIDS 20:1207-8 http://amedeo.com/lit.php?id=16691076

Ozawa, T (1997). Genetic and functional changes in mitochondria associated with aging. Physiol Rev. 77:425-464. [PubMed]

Palmer, NB. Salcedo, J. Miller AL. et al. (2003). Psychiatric and social barriers to HIV medication adherence in a triply diagnosed methadone population. AIDS Patient Care STDS 17(12):636-644

Pappas, MK. Halkitis, PN. (2011). Sexual risk taking and club drug use across three age cohorts of HIV-positive gay and bisexual men in New York City. AIDS Care.; 23:1410–6. [PMC free article] [PubMed]

Parekh, BS. Shaffer, N. Pau, C-P, et al. (1991) Lack of correlation between maternal antibodies to V3 Loop peptides of gp120 and perinatal HIV-1 transmission: the NYC Peri-Natal HIV Transmission Collaborative Study. AIDS 5:1179-1184

Patel, P. Hanson, DL. Sullivan, PS. (2008). Incidence of types of cancer among HIV-infected persons compared with the general population in the United States, 1992-2003. Ann Intern Med.;148 (10):728–736 [PubMed]

Pentamidine injection: Uses, Side Effects, Interaction, Pictures…(2017). Retrieved from https://www.web-md.com/drugs/2/drug-8687/pen-tamidine-injection/details

Pillard, RC. (1988). Sexual orientation and mental disorder. Psychiatric Annals 18(1):52-56

Pneumocystis pneumonia | Fungal Diseases (2017). CDC Retrieved from https://www.cdc.gov/fungal/diseases/pneumocystis-pneumonia/index.html

Portegies, P (2010). HIV/HAART and the brain—what's going on? J Int AIDS Soc.;13 (suppl 4):35

Quinn, TC. Wawer, MJ. Sewankambo, N. et al. (2000). Viral load and heterosexual transmission of human immunodeficiency virus type 1. Rakai Project Study Group. N Engl J Med.;342 (13):921-929. Available at: https://www.ncbi.nlm.nih.gov/pubmed/10738050.

Rabkin, JG. (1996). Prevalence of psychiatric disorders in HIV illness. Retrieved from https://www.ncbi.nlm.nih.gov/pmc/articles/PMC1160559/

Redfield, RR. Wright, DC. Tramont, EC. The Walter Reed staging classification for HTLV-III/LAV infection N Engl J Med 1986;314:131-2. [PubMed]

Riera, M La. Fuente, Ld. L, Castanyer, B. et al. (2002). [Adherence to antiretroviral therapy measured by pill count and drug serum concentrations Variables associated with a bad adherence.] Med Clin (Barc) 119(8):286-292.

Rollot, F. Nazal, EM. Chauvelot-Moachon, et al (2003). Tenofovir-related Fanconi syndrome with nephrogenic diabetes insipidus in a patient with acquired immunodeficiency syndrome: the role of lopinavir-ritonavir-didanosine. Clin Infect Dis 37: e174-6. http://amedeo.com/lit.php?id=14689363

R^ttgers, HR. Weltermann, BM. Evers, S. Husstedt, IW. (2000). Psychiatrische Akutsymptomatik als Erstmanifestation einer HIV-Infektion. Nervenarzt 71: 404-10. http://amedeo.com/lit.php?id=10846717

Saykin, AJ. Janssen, RS. Sprehn, GC. et al (1988). Neuropsychological dysfunction in HIV-infection: characterization in a lymphadenopathy cohort. International Journal of Clinical Neuropsychology 10(2):81-95

Schooley, RT. Merigan, TC. Gaut, P. et al (1990). Recombinant soluble CD4 therapy in patients with AIDS and ARC. Ann Intern Med 112: 247-53. http://amedeo.com/lit.php?id=2297203

Seth, D. Kamat, D. Montejo, J. DRESS (2008). syndrome: a practical approach for primary care practitioners. Clin Pediatr (Phila) ;47:947-52. [PubMed]

Sewell, DD. Jeste, DV. Atkinson, JH. Heaton, RK. Hesselink, JR. Wiley, C. et al. (1994). HIV-associated psychosis: a study of 20 cases. San Diego HIV Neurobehavioral Research Center Group. Am J Psychiatry; 151:237-42 [PubMed]

Siliciano, JD. Kajdas, J. Finzi, D. et al (2003). Long-term follow-up studies confirm the stability of the latent reservoir for HIV-1 in resting CD4+ T cells Nature Med 9:727-728. http://amedeo.com/lit.php?id=12754504

Sonnabend, J. Witkin, SS. Purtilo, DT. (1983). Acquired immunodeficiency syndrome, opportunistic infections, and malignancies in male homosexuals: A hypothesis of etiologic factors in pathogenesis. JAMA 249:23470-2374

Stebbing, J. Gazzard, B. & Douck, DC. (2004). Where does HIV live? New England Journal of medicine. 350(18):1872-80

Stramer, SL. (2003) Third reported US case of breakthrough HIV transmission from NAT screened blood. Transmission 43(Supplement):40A

Stringer, JR. Beard, CB. Miller, RF. Wakefield, AE. (2002). A new name (Pneumocystis jiroveci) for Pneumocystis from humans. Emerg Infect Dis 8:891-6. http://amedeo.com/lit.php?id=12194762

Structure and function of HIV-1 integrase. - NCBI - NIH (2004). Retrieved from syndrome (AIDS). Acta Neurology Scandinavica, 71(5):337-53.

The Discovery and Development of Antiretroviral Agents (2017). Retrieved from http://www.apps.who.int › All › Medicine Information and Evidence for Policy › Medicines Policy

The Facts About HIV and Diarrhea Symptoms Can Range from Mild to Life-threatening By James Myhre and Dennis Sifris, MD | Reviewed by a board-certified physician Updated February 18, 2018

The Global HIV/AIDS Epidemic (2017). The Henry J Kaiser Family Foundation Retrieved from https://www.kff.org/global-health-policy/fact-sheet/the-global-hivaids-epedemic/

The HIV Life Cycle | Understanding HIV/AIDS (2017). AIDSinfo Retrieved from https://aidsinfo.nih.gov/understanding-hiv-aids/fact-sheets/19/73/the-hiv-life-cycle

The Interagency Advisory Panel on Research Ethics (PRE) (2017). Retrieved from http://www.pre.ethics.gc.ca/eng/policy-politique/initiatives/tcps2-eptc2/chapter1.../ch1_en

Treisman, Glenn J. & Kaplina, Adam I. (1999). AIDS education for psychiatrists. Prim Psychiatry 6:71-73

Tsai, AC. Weiser, SD. Petersen, M. Ragland, K. Kushel, MB. Bangsberg, DR. (2010). A marginal structural model to estimate the causal effect of antidepressant medication treatment on viral suppression among homeless and marginally housed persons with HIV. Arch Gen Psychiatry. 67:1282-1290. [PMC free article] [PubMed]

Types of Research Methods (2008). Retrieved from http://www.archives.gadoe.org/.../Types.of.Research. Methods.SERVE%20Center pdf?p...Type=D

UNAIDS (2001): Guidelines for using HIV testing technologies in surveillance: selection, evaluation, and implementation. WHO/CDS/CSR/EDC/16

Understanding Descriptive and Inferential Statistics (2017). Laerd Statistics Retrieved from https://zt`tistics.laerd.com/statistical-guides/descriptive-inferentail-statistics U.S.

U.S. Federal Funding for HIV/AIDS: (2017). Trends Over Time | The Henry J...Retrieved from https://www.kff.org/global-health.../u-s-federal-funding-for-hivaids-trends-over-time/

Vance, DE. Ross, JA. Moneyham, L. Farr, KF. Fordham, P. (2010). A model of cognitive decline and suicidal ideation in adults aging with HIV. J Neurosci Nurs. 42:150–156. [PubMed]

Volberding, PA. Lagakos, SW. Koch, MA. et al (1990). Zidovudne in asymptomatic HIV infection. A controlled trial in persons with fewer than 500 CD4-positive cells per cubic millimeter. N Engl J Med 322:941-9 http://amedeo.com/lit.php?id=1969115

Walkup, J. Akincigil, A. Hoover, DR. Siege, l. MJ, Amin. S, Crystal S. (2011). Use of Medicaid data to explore community characteristics associated with HIV prevalence among beneficiaries with schizophrenia. Public Health Rep;126 (Suppl 3):89–101. [PMC free article] [PubMed]

Walzer, PD. Perl, DP. Krogstad, DJ. Rawson, PG. Schultz, MG. (1984). Pneumocystis carinii pneumonia in the United States: epidemiologic, diagnostic, and clinical features. Ann Intern Med; 80:83-93.

What are HIV and AIDS? (2017). AVERT Retrieved from https://www.avert.org › Information on HIV › About HIV & AIDS

Where did HIV come from? (2017). The AIDS ~Institute Retrieved from http://www.theaidsinstitute.org › EDUCATION › AIDS 101

What is a cohort study in medical research? (2016). Medical News Today Retrieved from https://www.medicalnewstoday.com/articles/281703.php What is RNA? | RNA Society (2017) Retrieved from https://www.rnasociety.org/about/what-is-rna/

Winston, A. Puls, R. Kerr, SJ. et al (2011). Dynamics of cognitive change in HIV-infected individuals commencing three different initial antiretroviral regimens: a randomized, controlled study. HIV Med. 13(4):245-251. [PubMed]

World Health Organization. Clinical practice guidelines. (1994). Washington DC: U.S. Department of Health and Human Services AHCPR Pub. #94-0592;14

Wutoh, AK. Elekwachi, O. Clarke-Tasker, V. Daftary, M. Powell, NJ. Campusano, G. Assessment (2003). And predictors of antiretroviral adherence in older HIV-infected patients. J Acquir Immune Defic Syndr. 33(Suppl 2): S106-S114. [PubMed]

Yun, LW. Maravi, M. Kobayashi, J. Barton, PL. Davidson, AJ. (2006). Antidepressant treatment improves adherence to antiretroviral therapy among depressed HIV-infected patients, J Acquir Immune Defic Syndr, vol. 41 (pg. 254-5)

Zou, S. Dorsey, KA. Notari, EP. et al. (2010). Prevalence, incidence, and residual risk of human immunodeficiency virus and hepatitis C virus infections among United States blood donors since the introduction of nucleic acid testing. Transfusion 50:1495-504.

www.ingramcontent.com/pod-product-compliance
Lightning Source LLC
LaVergne TN
LVHW041621060526
838200LV00040B/1382